Vascular Dementia
Sundown Dementia
and
Lewy Bodies Dementia

Stages, symptoms, signs, prognosis, diagnosis, treatments, progression, care and mood changes all covered.

By

Lyndsay Leatherdale

Thanks to my mum for being such a great mum. Even though she works long hours, she always has time to listen and help me. Her office door is always open to my sibling and I. She is an author herself and she inspired me to write this book.

In addition, my dad always supports mum and us kids in whatever we do. He's always there with an encouraging word and an understanding heart.

I also want to thank all the people who generously shared their personal experiences about living with dementia patients. I've learned so much from them and appreciate their openness and honesty.

Thanks goes to all the professionals in the field that I spoke to whose experience and knowledge helped me understand dementia.

Table of Contents

Foreword 9

A note to our readers in the UK 11

Chapter 1. Dementia in Today's Society 14

1. The Baby Boomers... 14

2. Growing older in America 16

3. Life Expectancy keeps going up 16

Chapter 2. Understanding Dementia........................ 18

1. What is Dementia... 18

2. Signs, Symptoms and Characteristics of Dementia................. 19

3. Difference between Dementia and Normal Memory Loss 21

4. Diagnosing Dementia 24

Chapter 3. Stages of Dementia 26

Chapter 4. Vascular Dementia 32

1. What is Vascular Dementia? 32

2. Signs, Symptoms and Characteristics of Vascular Dementia 33

3. Preventing Vascular Dementia 35

4. Reducing the Effects of Vascular Dementia............ 37

5.Caring for Someone with Vascular Dementia 39

Chapter 5. Sundown Dementia 43

1. What is Sundown Dementia?.................................. 43

2. Signs, Symptoms and Characteristics of Sundown Dementia... 47

3. Caring for Someone with Sundown Dementia 48

4. Shadowing 52

Chapter 6. Lewy Body Dementia 55

1. What is Lewy Bodies Dementia? 55

2. Signs, Symptoms and Characteristics of Lewy Bodies Dementia 56

3. Caring for Someone with Lewy Bodies Dementia.................. 58

Chapter 7. Other Manifestations of Dementia 61

1. Alzheimer's Disease... 61

2. Mixed dementia 61

3. Parkinson's Disease 62

4. Frontotemporal dementia 63

5. Creutzfeldt-Jacob disease 64

6. Normal Pressure Hydrocephalus 65

7. Huntington's disease 66

8. Wernicke-Korsakoff syndrome.................................... 66

9. Mild Cognitive Impairment (MCI)................................. 67

Chapter 8. Diabetes and Dementia 68

Chapter 9. Behavioural Changes Caused by Dementia............ 71

1. Causes of Behavioural Changes 71

2. Behaviour: Aggression 72

3. Behaviour: Wandering... 73

4. Behaviour: Sexual Behaviours.................................... 74

5. Behaviour: Screaming... 74

6. Behaviour: Self-Harming.. 75

7. Behaviour: Resistiveness 75

8. Behaviour: Hoarding... 76

9. Behaviour: Catastrophic Reactions.............................. 77

10. Behaviour: Repetitive Actions 77

11. Managing Behavioural Changes 78

Chapter 10. Medical Problems Associated with Dementia 80

Table of Contents

1. Causes of Medical Problems 80

2. Medical Problem: Psychosis 81

3. Medical Problem: Sleep Disturbances 82

4. Medical Problem: Jerking Movements 83

5. Medical Problem: Constipation 84

6. Medical Problem: Agnosia 85

7. Medical Problem: Pressure Sores 85

8. Medical Problem: Loss of Mobility 86

9. Medical Problem: Poor Dental Health 86

10. Medical Problem: Fits 87

11. Managing Medical Problems 87

Chapter 11. Mood Changes Caused by Dementia 89

1. Mood Change: Apathy 89

2. Mood Change: Loneliness 90

3. Mood Change: Boredom 90

4. Mood Change: Depression 91

5. Mood Change: Anxiety 91

6. Managing Mood Changes 92

Chapter 12. Case Studies of Dementia 94

1. Case Study Number One: Amy's Mum 94

2. Case Study Number Two: My Grandmother 100

Chapter 13. When Additional Care is Needed 110

1. Where to keep your Patient...................................110

2. Keeping the patient in her own home 111

3. Are you going to be her caregiver?.......................112

4. Telling Your Loved One She Needs Help 113

Table of Contents

Chapter 14. Providing Care as a Family..................... 115

1. Safety Devices 115

2. Infections 116

3. Falls 117

4. Burns or scalding 119

5. Choking, cuts, and poisoning.................................120

6. Fire hazards and Prevention 121

7. Finding Time for Yourself 122

Chapter 15. Aids and Devises for Care...................... 123

1. GPS Trackers 123

2. Memory Aids...125

3. Date Clocks and Calendars 125

4. Programmed Phones 126

5. Telecare Alarms..127

Chapter 16. Caring for a Patient with Dementia.................. 129

1. Personal Care 129

2. Mobility Care 133

3. Nutritional Care...135

4. Daily Chores 137

5. Companionship 137

Chapter 17. Remedies for Dementia 139

1. Coconut Oil 139

2. Vitamin D and Vitamin D3 141

3. Herbal Treatments 142

4. Magnetic Fields 143

5. A word about medication 144

Table of Contents

Chapter 18. Finding outside Care **145**

  Types of Outside Care **145**

  1. Option One: In-Home Care..**146**
    Choosing an In-Home Care Agency 147
    What does an Agency Offer 150
    Cost of Hiring From an Agency..152
    Cost of Hiring a Private Caregiver 153

  2. Option Two: Live-In Care **154**
    Choosing a Live-In Caregiver 156
    Cost of Hiring a Live-In Caregiver 157

  3. Option Three: Nursing Home Care.....................................**158**
    Choosing an Nursing Home...159
    Cost of a Nursing Home 161

Chapter 19. What you can do to help.................................. **163**

Chapter 20. UK Options and Costs for Dementia Care........... **165**

  1. Demographics in the UK **165**

  2. Cost of Care in the UK...**167**

  3. Frequently Asked Questions (FAQs) Regarding Costs **168**

  4. Care at Home **173**

Chapter 21. Resources and References.................................. **174**

  1. Family Support Resources...**174**

  2. U.S. Specific Care Resources **175**

  3. UK Specific Care Resources **175**

  4. References **176**

Foreword

Dementia. For many people, dementia is often thought of as an illness of the old. For many, dementia is not something that affects people who have succumbed to Alzheimer's and not something that the average person experiences, if they are not genetically predisposed to it. Unfortunately, this is not the case and anyone, regardless of family history, can be affected with some type of dementia or another.

Dementia is a silent disease that affects thousands of people every year. It can start suddenly or it can develop over time but for all, the effects are devastating to the families of and to the people living with the disease.

I will describe three forms of dementia, their suspected causes, and the tips for caregivers and families, but to start, I want to stress the difference between dementia and Alzheimer's.

Dementia is an impairment in the terms of how the brain functions and how memory is utilized. It interferes with a person's ability to function on a day-to-day basis.

Alzheimer's is also a deterioration of the mind and it is a disease that affects memory and the brains working functions. It is a degenerative condition that worsens over time and is fatal.

While it may seem the same, the main difference between the two is that Alzheimer's is a form of dementia, while the term dementia is an umbrella term used to describe a number of different types of dementia. It is important to note that dementia can occur without the presence of Alzheimer's and it can be caused by a number of known and unknown factors, which we will discuss later in this book.

The aim of this book is to bring light to a topic that is often kept in the dark, seeing as it touches on so many emotions.

One question that I often get asked is how I became interested in the topic of dementia and why, even at a young age, I have acquired so much information about the disease. The answer lies in my own personal experience, which I would like to share with you before we look at the individual dementias in this book.

****

It was a devastating blow when my grandmother was diagnosed with dementia. Not because my family and I had thought we were impervious to such a thing but because my grandmother had gone from a vibrant and extremely strong woman to one that was unsure and faded in a matter of only a few weeks.

At 86 years old, no one in the family had thought much about the routine tests that were scheduled for her. She had spent her life as an outgoing individual. She loved to travel, was constantly on the go and was spending her twilight years enjoying herself to the fullest. The only shadow on her perfect life in Belgium was an irregular heartbeat that had bothered her for over 30 years.

That was the reason for the tests, to determine if there was a hidden condition that could affect her health. Her doctor, or GP as we refer to them in the UK, referred her to a heart-specialist who suggested a series of injections.

The injections, we were told, were nothing to be worried about and on the day of the procedure, it didn't cross anyone's mind to do so. Unfortunately, my grandmother quickly developed a hematoma, which is a localized collection of blood outside the blood vessel. The hematoma had developed under the skin where the injection was given, in her stomach area.

The sudden hematoma sent her into a coma and when she finally woke up, she had developed vascular dementia. The vibrant woman that had showered me with love as a child was gone and my family was left to wonder why.

From the moment my grandmother was diagnosed with dementia, I saw that it was putting a big strain on my mum, who was constantly worrying about her mum (my grandmother). I came to understand the challenges that my family were facing. My grandmother lives in Belgium and we lived in the UK so that made everything even more difficult for my mum and for myself as I was asked to help out on numerous occasions.

As I am a Neuro Science student, I was very interested in how dementia would affect my grandmother and my family. In my education, I have focused on the study of the brain, specifically in the area of psychology.

This gave me the inclination to write this book. I wanted to look after my grandmother as much as I could and I would go with her to every doctor's visit and hospital appointments. I spoke to nurses, caregivers, doctors, other people who had dementia patients in their families, etc.. I now understand the journey that so many families face when a loved one develops dementia. It is not my aim to focus on medical terminology and diagnosis in this book, as I am not a doctor, but more to give practical information, once a patient has been diagnosed as dementia.

A note to our readers in the UK

We can all appreciate that dementia is free from boarders and can traverse the oceans that separate the world. Everyone, in any country or continent, can experience the emotion of a loved one with dementia. The patients, wherever they are, suffer the disease in the same unfortunate manner. All experience the same issues that are linked to the signs, symptoms, and behaviors and there is no difference according to demographics between the UK and the USA.

The majority of this book addresses the families of patients in many different countries equally, although we have focused on the USA and the UK. In this book, wherever we provide costs and resources for the U.S. reader, we do the same towards the end in a chapter solely for readers in the UK. It is important to note that when we address treatments and steps towards dealing with dementia, when there is no monetary breakdown, it is applicable to any location, even outside the two countries that are the main focus. We know that the UK reader will get the same benefits from this book as their U.S. counterparts.

In this book, we will examine the full range of consequences that dementia brings for all concerned. If you have a parent, relative, or partner who is showing signs of dementia, we hope that you find our information practical and relevant to your needs.

We will be discussing the different types of dementia with particular emphasis on Vascular, Sundown, and Lewy Bodies Dementia. We focus on the progression of dementia, how dementia affects the behaviour of the people diagnosed with it, and most importantly, we look at the best way to care for these people.

We will detail the pitfalls and bumps in the care giving road; outlining, at times abrasively, the harshness and difficulties involved.

Most importantly, we hope you will sense the depth with which we treat the various subjects, particularly those revolving around managing the disease and care giving.

We have covered various practical approaches that can be applied to care if you intend to provide hands-on care yourself. We cover a discussion of the hazards that patients of dementia face when living in their own home and how to make it a possibility for them with the least amount of risk.

If you are thinking of hiring caregivers, we have also covered the many different angles to hiring so it becomes an easier task for you. Finally, we will discuss what to expect from institutions such as assisted living facilities and care homes if you are considering these and other long-term options.

All the patients with dementia are referred to as "the patient" or "patient" since sufferers can be male or female. In addition, when we refer to them as a pronoun, the patient with dementia is always referred to as a she. It is important to note that we are not implying that dementia does not affect men but using one pronoun makes discussing dementia much clearer.

In addition, whenever we refer to a physician or doctor in a pronoun, it is done using the "he" pronoun. Again, we are not implying that physicians are always male but it is to make a clearer separation between patient – she – and doctor – he.

Although we are using a universal and general term, we hope that we can connect with you on an individual basis. We hope that you can relate to the information we are giving you and that you can share your own experiences while reading.

We know the trials and tribulations involved with being a caregiver, especially when the patient with dementia is a loved one. We also know that every experience is different and no one can truly fathom what you are going through as a caregiver. We do hope, however, that you'll find some degree of solace in these pages and with that solace a small measure of understanding, support and consolation.

Chapter 1. Dementia in Today's Society

Before we begin an in depth look at dementia, it is important to really understand dementia as it is in today's society. At no other time in our history have we been faced with the problem of dementia in the scale that we are about to face it in the next few decades.

In fact, dementia is one of the leading diseases that are affecting our elderly each year and there seems to be no sign of it stopping. Currently, there are over 24.5 million people living with dementia. In addition, 4.6 million new cases of dementia occur every year.

With these alarming rates, it is clear that we are heading towards an epidemic of enormous proportions and it is directly related to how our population is aging.

In this chapter, I will go over the many factors that are leading to this crisis that is just on the horizon.

1. The Baby Boomers

People mostly referred to it as the "double whammy," although it has also been called the "vortex". If you combine a whirlwind with a large, twirling funnel, you get a vortex into which people are sucked. That is exactly what is happening to our population.

But rewind for a moment to 60 years ago. This was a time in our history when there was a sudden influx or "boom" to our population. Families were much larger for several decades and it was not unheard of for families to have 6 or more children. Although there was a viable reason for larger families during that time period, what was not taken into consideration was the fact that that population will eventually age.

By the turn of the millennium, the boomers born in the late 1940s were entering into their early 50's in large numbers. They were typically at, or near, the peak of their careers. In addition, many of them were faced with a myriad of responsibilities; from aging parents to grown children. Suddenly, this population found themselves stretched thin.

They frequently saw their lives unravelling when one of their care giving parents died, leaving the other parent at risk, or when a previously independent 80 year-old parent fell and broke a hip. Or when something traumatic, a stroke perhaps, caused a perfectly self-sustaining man to succumb to an onslaught of dementia and total dependence.

In many of those cases where a sudden illness occurred, the 50-year olds with kids of college age suddenly found themselves grappling with the twirling funnel of the vortex that I described earlier in this chapter.

Although many of these baby boomers were men faced with the role of a dual caregiver, research has shown that it has predominantly been the women who did the heavy lifting. Research shows that in 4 out of 5 households, even when the suddenly impaired was the parent of the alpha male of the house, it has been the women who had to drop everything –put a hold on all facets of their lives- and run to the rescue of the aging parent, for the aging parent could not be left unattended, not even for 10 minutes. That road far too often led to women suffering from exhaustion, stress and self-neglect.

With children of college age, and with aging parents who, not uncharacteristically, frequently outlived their resources, many 50-year olds also found themselves staring at the dismal prospect of having to spend lifelong savings.

It is this sudden need for instant care giving that has caused a crisis for many families and it is quickly becoming a cultural drain on our own social programs.

2. Growing older in America

As I have mentioned, the "double whammy" of caring for aging parents is a predicament that many families are currently facing. It has been described by Laura Carstensen, Director of the Stanford Center on Longevity:

"The norms that told us when to get an education, when to marry, when to retire evolved when we lived half as long as now; In today's norms, we're raising kids, reaching the peak of our careers, and taking care of aging parents, all at the same time."

Experts say the number of adult children taking care of their parents will increase as people live longer.

According to a 2011 study done by MetLife Mature Market Institute for the U.S., there are nearly 10 million people over the age of 50 who care for their parents. That figure has more than tripled over the past 15 years.

According to the U.S. Department of Health and Human Services, the demand for informal caregivers (family, friends and neighbours) is expected to grow by more than 20 percent in the next 15 years as baby boomers age.

3. Life Expectancy keeps going up

Along with the increasing statistics on aging and dementia, one statistic is actually having a profound impact on the quality of life for baby boomers and their children. That statistic is life expectancy.

In the U.S., life expectancy is going up incredulously. The National Institute of Aging says that by 2040, life expectancy for men will be 86 and for women 91. Here is the take-away on that from two different angles, the demographic, and the financial:

For the demographic take, Dr. Jennifer N. Brok says in *'The Evolution of the Aging Population'*: *"10,000 baby boomers entering the Medicare age every day, heralding a seismic shift in demographics worldwide. By 2020, there will be 115 million seniors in America."*

Dr. Brok refers to it as the seismic shift in demographics. It has also been referred to as the "demographic time bomb" and "tidal wave" of older people, the inference being that this wave will be accompanied by massive governmental incompetence and lack of resources.

And here is how people might end up coping with that according to Rd. Ken Dychtwald, Ph.D. in Gerontology and sought-after public speaker who says: *"...for others, this 'longevity bonus' will be fraught with pain and suffering. Large numbers of tomorrow's elders could wind up impoverished, left stranded by an absence of financial preparedness and dwindling old age entitlements."*

As you can see, the aging population will create many problems for both the families who are affected and for society as a whole.

Chapter 2. Understanding Dementia

Before we move on to the actual care and needs of patients, family members and friends with dementia, it is important to truly understand what dementia actually is.

Often, when we think of dementia, we think of how it is depicted in movies or on television. The sudden loss of memory and the unusual behavior that can be both endearing and funny; however, there is nothing endearing or funny about dementia.

As a result of this depiction in mainstream media, there is rarely a true foundation for people to base their understanding on and it can be crippling when faced with a family member with dementia. At times, it can be a sudden occurrence and at other times it can be a gradual progression. Regardless of how it manifests, dementia is a serious disease that can greatly affect the quality of life for both you and your loved one.

In this chapter, I will discuss the many different things that you should know regarding dementia so that you have a basis of understanding before we begin to look at dementia in several of its different manifestations.

1. What is Dementia

When we look at dementia in a simplified way, it is a disease that affects the brain and causes both memory loss and cognitive decline.

Dementia is a progressive disease, which means that it continues to get worse over time. In addition, dementia is not memory loss due to age, which is completely normal. Later in this chapter, I will go over the factors of normal memory loss so you are aware of the differences.

18

With dementia, the decline of cognitive abilities is often linked to other problems including emotional stress and a loss of control. Dementia continually progresses to a steady decline in cognitive function, however, some forms of dementia, if they are caught early, can be treated.

In fact, some forms of dementia can be reversed as long as the prognosis is made in the early stages of the disease. If it is not caught, the disease is more difficult to reverse and in the majority of cases, nothing can be done but to improve the quality of life for a loved one as the disease progresses.

2. Signs, Symptoms and Characteristics of Dementia

When a family is faced with dementia, one of the first things that I recommend is to understand the signs, symptoms and characteristics of dementia. Later in this book, I will go over the different forms of dementia and look at the many different symptoms that are prevalent in that form, however, for now, it is important to look at the general symptoms.

One thing that you should be aware of, is that dementia is a number of symptoms that can also be linked to natural aging and other conditions. It is important to understand these differences and to also contact a medical professional when you suspect that the symptoms may be something more.

In addition, it is important to understand that one symptom does not pinpoint the cause as being dementia. Dementia is a collection of symptoms. What this means, is that it affects several areas of the person including the intellectual functioning, memory and even personality. All of these symptoms create a strain on relationships and interfere with the patient's ability to function in a positive and constructive manner.

For many with dementia, the symptoms and signs often start off in a slow manner. There may only be a few indicators or characteristics that alert caregivers and these can be as simple as the following:

- Using the wrong word to describe something or someone

- Difficulty following instructions or directions given to them

- Asks the same question or questions repeatedly

- Forgets about personal hygiene

- Forgets to eat

- Seems to disregard personal safety

- Forgets routine tasks

- Seems disoriented in familiar places and unsure of dates

Many times, when those first characteristics begin to manifest themselves, it is easy to overlook them. After all, everyone has experienced times when they have been forgetful; however, these problems will continue to compound. Very quickly, these problems begin to emerge in a pattern that leaves many caregivers aware that the problem is more than just normal aging.

In addition to those indicators, caregivers will see a number of different symptoms and signs. These can include, but are not limited to:

- Memory loss

- Problems with balance

- Inability to communicate, both verbally and physically

- Problems with gait and walking

- Problems with motor control

- Neglect of personal care

- Impaired judgement concerning personal safety

- Paranoia

- Agitation

- Hallucinations

- Inappropriate behavior

- Disorientation

- Inability to process abstract ideas

3. Difference between Dementia and Normal Memory Loss

As you know, I have already mentioned that some of the signs of dementia can merely be a normal process of aging. Memory loss, disorientation and being forgetful are very normal as long as it is occasional and not constant. In fact, studies have shown that a gradual memory loss after the age of 40 can be normal for many people due to the brain shrinking slowly with age.

What is not normal is when there is memory loss or cognitive loss that is sudden, severe and progressing rapidly. This is when you should be concerned that something more serious than natural memory loss has occurred.

With normal memory loss, you will be looking at the following symptoms and signs.

- *Decreased ability to problem solve.* Again, this should be a slow progression if it is commonly associated with aging. It takes longer to figure out a problem that is presented.

- *Slower cognitive ability.* Although learning, reaction times and accessing memories can be affected by aging, it is generally just a slow down and not an inability to access those cognitive abilities. In addition, you may need hints and cues to help remember things.

- *Decreased Ability to Concentrate.* Generally, this means that you can be distracted easier, which can actually affect your cognitive abilities and your ability to learn.

Although I focused on aging as it would affect an individual, it is usually the caregiver that notices the affects of normal memory loss. In addition, it is usually the caregivers that notice the signs of dementia before the patient actually realizes it.

To give you some understanding of what the difference between normal memory loss and dementia is when you are observing it, here are some examples:

Example Number One:

Normal Memory Loss:

- Is at a loss for words occasionally or appears to have to search for a word when talking.

Dementia:

- Substitutes words for other words or frequently searches for the right word.

Example Number Two:

Normal Memory Loss:

- Has difficulty when remembering directions but does not become lost when in a familiar location.

Dementia:

- Becomes disoriented and lost in a familiar place. May have difficulty determining the difference between a familiar place and a strange place.

Example Number Three:

Normal Memory Loss:

- Complains about being forgetful but when asked to describe instances, is able to give examples of when he was forgetful.

Dementia:

- Complains about being forgetful but when asked to describe instances, is unable to give examples of when he was forgetful.

Example Number Four:

Normal Memory Loss:

- Remembers important events but may be forgetful of regular events or low impact events. In addition, the patient remembers recent events and can converse about them.

Dementia:

- Unable to remember both important and low impact events. Patients can recall events from long term memory but are unable to recall and converse about recent events.

Example Number Five:

Normal Memory Loss:

- Interacts with people in much of the same ways as before. No loss of interpersonal social skills.

Dementia:

- Inappropriate behavior in social situations and there is a decline in interest for social interactions.

As you can see, in some ways it can be hard to determine the difference between normal memory loss and dementia, as some of the signs mirror the others. However, what you can also see is that some areas are impacted more severely and it is those areas that you want to pay close attention to.

Normal memory loss that is associated with aging is not something to be worried about. If it becomes more serious and you start to see one or two signs or symptoms of dementia, then it is important to seek medical help for your loved one.

4. Diagnosing Dementia

Diagnosing dementia is not something that should be done by a caregiver or a family member. Dementia needs to be properly diagnosed by a trained physician, be it your family doctor or a specialist.

One thing that caregivers should do in the process of diagnosing dementia is to document any instances where the patient's seems to be exhibiting a sign of dementia. Having this concrete documentation before the doctor's appointment will give the physician a better understanding of how the dementia has been progressing and the steps needed to take for adequate treatment.

When diagnosing dementia, the physician will ask for a complete medical history of the patient. This will include health problems such as high blood pressure, heart problems and even cognitive problems. In addition, family history, including the occurrence of depression in both the family and the patient will be needed.

Once the history of the patient is determined, the physician will go over the symptoms and signs that have been observed. As I have mentioned, it is important to have the dates documented as well as the progression of the symptoms as the physician will want to use this evidence in diagnosis.

Once there is a clear picture of the patient's history, tests are done to determine the cause of the cognitive problems. The first is often blood work and other laboratory tests that help determine whether there is a metabolic condition that could be impairing proper cognitive functioning. In addition, vitamin deficiencies are often ruled out.

Next, a neurological exam is often done to determine neurological function. In some cases, after things have been ruled out, brain imaging will be done, again, to check how the brain is functioning. Finally, a mental status test, or neuropsychological test, is performed.

Once all these tests are administered, the physician will have a clearer image of whether the patient has dementia and usually the type of dementia that he has.

In most cases, the brain of the patient will also be scanned.

Chapter 3. Stages of Dementia

Before we get into the different types of dementia that can occur, it is important to understand a bit more about dementia in general. Specifically, the stages of dementia are something that should be discussed, as this can greatly affect quality of life and how a caregiver will administer care.

One thing that I want to note is that dementia often occurs in stages. It is a progressive disease, which means that it continually becomes worse as the patient ages. What is also important to note is that not all dementia progresses through the same stages and most do not progress at the same speed. In fact, some can progress very quickly and it can often appear as though some stages are missed.

Another point is that the first few stages of dementia are often overlooked. In many cases, dementia is first noticed during the third stage and that is why it often seems to progress rapidly.

When looking at the stages, we are actually describing seven different stages. The first four stages are often grouped together and are viewed as less severe cases of dementia. Many times it is during the first four stages that steps can be taken to reverse or delay the effects of the disease.

The final three stages are the more severe and are often described under the Global Deterioration Scale for Assessment of Primary Degenerative Dementia, also known as The Resiberg Scale. We will go over each stage so you, as a caregiver, will have a greater understanding of the progression of dementia. However, later in this book, we will discuss the care needed, in relation to the stages.

Stage One: Slight Memory Loss

During the first stage of dementia, there are only slight indicators that there is a problem. The first stage is often confused with normal memory loss that is commonly caused by aging.

One of the very first things that occur is when the memory begins to "play up". Commonly used words are forgotten and it can take some effort and time for the patient to remember the word. During these moments of forgetfulness, you may see the patient becoming very embarrassed or frustrated.

These feelings can often lead to some behavioural changes including the patient becoming irritable. She may avoid speaking to people when there are direct questions involved and she may become withdrawn.

Another sign that you will see is confabulation. This is when the patient begins to create stories in order to fill gaps that are occurring in her recollections. Although the first few times she uses confabulation, she may be aware of the lies, as she progresses through stage one, the stories she has made up become as real as a memory.

Stage Two: Confusion and Disorientation

During stage two, the symptoms from stage one will still be present. Memory loss is still occurring and confabulation will also be occurring, usually on a more frequent basis.

In addition to those signs, the patient may begin to withdraw from society. There is almost an appearance of being more relaxed and they spend more of their time focusing on past experiences.

Another change that you often see during stage two is confusion in speech patterns. At times, phrases the patient uses are not as clear and they can be muddled. In addition, the patient may start a sentence in mid thought or shift around in a thought so their speech becomes broken and incoherent.

During the second stage, the patient will also begin to be distracted easily when following directions or doing simple tasks. An example of this is picking up a pair of glasses and remembering that she had to get them to get the mail but then forgetting why she has her glasses. She may even forget what to do with her glasses.

Lastly, the second stage of dementia often brings disorientation and confusion with people. The patient will begin to confuse people with others, even if the people she confuses them for are deceased. This is a very difficult time for caregivers since being confused for someone else can be painful, especially if they are a close family member.

Stage Three: Withdrawal to the Past

Stage three is often the stage where family members begin to realize that something is wrong with the patient. Small moments of confusion are easily overlooked; however, in stage three, these moments occur more frequently and often last longer.

During this stage, patients with dementia start to withdraw even further into the past and become so preoccupied with their memories that they live almost entirely in that time and reality.

Attached with this reality is an inability to truly communicate their needs. In fact, some may rely less on communicating through language and will rely more on expressing through body language. This can be very confusing for a caregiver as some needs, wants and even feelings can be overlooked.

Most verbal communication is done with either a "yes" or "no" answer or the caregiver may need to use words that have meaning to the patient in relation to their past.

Another problem that can occur during this stage is wandering. When this happens, it is important to know that there is usually a valid reason. Either the person is looking for something or someone, or is trying to prevent boredom.

Lastly, the patient may become incontinent during stage three; however, it does not occur with every patient.

Stage Four: Withdrawal from Society

During stage four, patients withdraw even further from the outside world. In fact, many patients will withdraw completely at this stage. They will often sit in a chair or in a bed and will not respond when other people come into the room.

They also have a very difficult time communicating and may not communicate in any way, including through body language. However, it is important to remember that while they may not be communicating to the caregiver, the caregiver is communicating to the patient. It is important to give the patient love, patience and perseverance through words, body language, tone, and touching so they continue to understand how important and cared for they are.

Stage Five: Pronounced Memory Loss

With pronounced memory loss, the patient has severe memory loss. She may have no idea of the present reality and will often become confused and alarmed by things that should be ordinary for her.

During this stage, she will need to have more aid from her caregivers and when you see this progression of memory loss; steps may need to be taken to ensure that she receives the proper care, such as through assisted living.

Although there is no guarantee on how long a stage will last, most cases of stage five last about 1 to 1 and a half years before it becomes worse.

Stage Six: Repetitive Behaviours

During this stage, the patient will become more agitated than she was previously. In addition, you may start to see repetitive behaviours, such as repeatedly pinching fluff off of a piece of clothing.

In addition, her overall ability to take care of herself will be greatly diminished, if not gone all together. Patients in stage six are usually incontinent and need a caregiver for even the most basic care.

Patients with this stage of dementia have a difficult time conversing and are often unable to speak at all. They have severe personality changes and may even begin to have delusions.

In addition, the inability to remember recent events become more frequent and patients with stage six often forget close family members or confuse them for other people.

Again, there is no guarantee on the number of years a person will stay in stage six, however, usually it lasts between 2 to 2 and a half years.

Stage Seven: Loss of Motor Skills

In this final stage of dementia, the patient will have lost both communication skills and motor skills. Usually the patient will be completely incontinent and will also need to rely on other methods of transportation.

During this stage, the patient needs 24 hour care and often caregivers must decide on the best possible care for the patient, usually including hospitalization.

Like many other stages, there is no guarantee for how long this stage lasts but generally, the stage lasts for 2 to 2 and a half years.

As I have mentioned, the prognosis for dementia is not good, especially if it has not been caught in time. For those who suffer through all seven stages of dementia, the disease is terminal and it is a hard journey for anyone who cares for the patient.

Chapter 4. Vascular Dementia

Now that we have gone through the stages and characteristics of dementia, it is time to look at the many different types of dementia that can occur. In this book, I am focusing on three types of dementia but later on, I will briefly go over the other forms of dementia.

If you remember from the foreword, vascular dementia is a condition that has touched me personally. My own grandmother had vascular dementia and sundown dementia combined and her care, which for a large part fell to me, was not a very pleasant experience at times. Much of the care guides in this book, as well as the whole reason for writing this book, comes down to my experience of working with a loved one diagnosed with vascular dementia and sundown dementia.

1. What is Vascular Dementia?

Vascular dementia is one of the more common manifestations of dementia. It is characterized by a sudden decline in memory and cognitive function that tapers off to a stable period before there is another sudden decline. However, it can also be characterized by the same gradual decline that we discussed in the stages of dementia.

Vascular dementia occurs when blood stops flowing to the brain for any reason including trauma. The brain gets its supply of Oxygen and nutrients through the blood, and if that is interrupted, even for a few seconds, brain cells will begin to die. An interruption of the blood flow to the brain can happen as a result of trauma to the brain, a stroke, a diseased vascular system or weakness and other factors, such as severe blood loss.

32

Another cause of vascular dementia is when the brain is deprived of blood flow due to small strokes or "silent" strokes–small, usually undiagnosed strokes known as TIAs "transient ischemic attacks". These strokes have a cumulative effect, over time, to cause the blood supply to be decreased to the brain, which results in a choking of the brain. When this occurs, the type of vascular dementia that occurs is known as multi-infarct dementia.

Another cause of vascular dementia can be blood clots that are either loose in the bloodstream or clogging the blood stream. Hypertension and high blood pressure are also causes of vascular dementia and it is linked to nearly 50% of all cases of the disease.

Lastly, lupus and temporal arteritis, both of which are autoimmune inflammatory diseases, have attributed to a smaller number of vascular dementia diseases but are another cause of the disease.

2. Signs, Symptoms and Characteristics of Vascular Dementia

Although vascular dementia has symptoms that are particular to it, its progression is in many ways similar to those of dementia, which I have already discussed. However, some of the symptoms, signs or characteristics that you may see are as follows:

- Depression, anxiety, and periods of utter confusion

- Incontinence

- Rapid decline in motor skills

- Dizziness, balance issues, weakness and paralysis

- Symptoms of a stroke

- Tremors

- Seizures

- Memory problems

- Problems relevant to the speed of thinking

- Concentration issues

- Communication issues

- Hallucinations and delusions

In addition to those signs and characteristics, many caregivers notice behavioural symptoms in the patients. These symptoms include:

- Difficulty when recalling words and communicating

- Disoriented even in very familiar surroundings

- Out-of-place expressions of laughter, crying out, or making other sounds

- Inability to function or to perform common tasks

- Inability to comply with instructions or to form judgments

It is important to note that vascular dementia affects every patient differently. In addition, the progression of vascular dementia differs greatly from person to person and the care that they need will also differ.

Some symptoms may be similar to those of other types of dementia and usually reflect increased difficulty to perform everyday activities such as eating, dressing, or shopping.

Unlike other dementias, vascular disease can thrust the patient into the advanced stages almost instantly. Its abruptness and degeneration depend, to a large extent, on the severity of the trauma the brain received. If the lack of blood supply to the brain was massive –as in more than for a few seconds- for example as a result of a significant stroke, the onslaught of the disease is immediate and significant.

If, on the other hand, the disease was acquired as a result of TIA, or silent strokes over the course of a significant amount of time, then the disease will manifest itself gradually, in which case it is likely to resemble other forms of dementia at first.

Regardless of the rate of advance, vascular dementia typically progresses in declines followed by stability before a further lapse is seen.

3. Preventing Vascular Dementia

Although vascular dementia is not always preventable, there are a few things that can be done to help avoid the disease.

Tip Number One: Check your Blood Pressure

First, always be aware of your blood pressure and make sure that it remains at a normal rate for your age, sex and weight. If you find that it is too high, follow the advice of your doctor to ensure that it is lowered.

Tip Number Two: Don't Smoke

Since smoking can create problems with blood flow, including blood clots, it is better if you do not smoke. If you do smoke, you should quit as soon as possible to help lower the risk of vascular dementia.

Tip Number Three: Control your Cholesterol

Another area of your health that you should watch is your cholesterol. Keeping it in a healthy range will ensure that you have a better vascular system and that will reduce the risk of vascular dementia.

Tip Number Four: Remove Salt from your Diet

Salt can cause a number of different health problems, including the hardening of arteries, so it is important to limit the amount of salt in your diet. This will help with blood flow and will reduce the risk of vascular dementia caused by silent strokes.

Tip Number Five: Exercise Daily

As everyone knows, exercise is one of the most important factors in caring for your health. Daily exercise will help to reduce your cholesterol levels and your blood pressure and this will reduce the risk of vascular dementia.

Generally, leading a healthier lifestyle will affect both your short term and long term health. Even if there are signs of vascular dementia occurring, it is important to note that switching your lifestyle or your patient's lifestyle could greatly improve the quality of life experienced.

4. Reducing the Effects of Vascular Dementia

Before we look at ways to reduce the effects of vascular dementia, I firstly wanted to look at vascular dementia as something that can be treated.

To begin, it is important to note that one out of ten cases of vascular dementia have been proven to be temporary in nature. In addition, in one case out of every ten diagnoses of vascular dementia, the effects of dementia have been completely reversed.

These cases may range from seriously adverse medical conditions, such as benign brain and other tumors, to malnutrition. Nutritional deficiencies, particularly with patients who are in institutions, are known to have disorientation and memory loss, both of which are possible symptoms of dementia. With proper nutrition, those symptoms have not only be lessened but also reversed.

However, any caregiver going into a treatment plan or management plan must remember that these cases are rare. In addition, while someone can suffer from vascular dementia, they can also suffer from a factor known as mixed dementia where more than one manifestation of dementia is present.

As a result, it is unclear how often the origins of dementia track back to vascular problems. Some estimates have it that vascular dementia may account for one-tenth to one-third of all cases of dementia. Furthermore, about one-fifth of people with Alzheimer's disease may also be suffering from vascular dementia. So, extrapolating from that, roughly 1.5 to 2 million people suffer from vascular dementia.

As you can see, vascular dementia is prevalent in a large population base and it is very important for both a caregiver and patient to take steps to improve the prognosis. While I am looking at the tips in relation to someone with vascular dementia, it is important to also follow the tips as a caregiver.

Tip Number One: Stick to a Routine

A day-to-day routine is very important for anyone who has dementia and if you are diagnosed with dementia, it is important to create your own routine. Do regular activities in a set order every day. By doing this, you will be able to keep your mind in the present. Lastly, it will help anyone suffering from vascular dementia feel balanced and will also stimulate their memory.

Tip Number Two: Be Patient

One of the most important tips that you can take to heart is to be patient. This means that you should take your time doing any task, especially if they are multipart, such as taking out the garbage.

In addition, try to avoid becoming frustrated with yourself. Remember that you will forget occasionally but if you take tasks slowly, find time to relax and reduce your frustration; you will find that the dementia does not affect you as much as it could.

Tip Number Three: Find Ways to Remember

Whether it is a note pad that you carry with you or post it notes that you leave around the house, it is important to have ways to remember things. Make sure that you update it daily and that you always have a list of your errands written down.

In addition, important dates, phone numbers and other information should be written down and placed in easy to find places. In doing this, you will ensure that you remember things much easier.

Tip Number Four: Reduce Distractions

As you know, distractions play a large part in causing confusion and disorientation so it is important to minimize them. Keep the television off when there is something you need to do. In addition, reduce clutter in your home and other things that could distract you. Lastly, take instructions in small steps. Don't have long instructions that can be distracting and lead you to being confused.

Tip Number Five: Communicate

Lastly, make sure that you take the time to communicate your needs with your caregivers. They need as many cues as possible to help you and you should openly give them.
Always make sure that you ask people to speak slower if you are having problems understanding them and don't hesitate to ask them to repeat things for you.
It can be a challenge to follow these steps but by doing so, you will have reduced the rate that vascular dementia controls you.

5.Caring for Someone with Vascular Dementia

Later in this book we will go over the general care of anyone suffering from dementia, however, there are some steps that you can do to make caring for someone with vascular dementia much easier.

The very first thing that you should remember, is that caring for someone with any form of dementia can be very stressful. It is very important to be aware of your own feelings as you care for anyone with vascular dementia so you are less likely to burn out.

When you are caring for a person with vascular dementia, try following these steps:

One: Keep Calendars and Clocks Out

The first thing that you should do when you are caring for someone with vascular dementia is to provide them with a link to the "here and now". Calendars and clocks are the perfect tool for this and something that you should keep out where they can see.

It may not seem like much, but these tools can help people with vascular dementia, and any form of dementia, reorient themselves to the present.

Two: Provide Activities

Another helpful tip to follow is to provide activities for your loved one who has been diagnosed with vascular dementia. The main reason for this is to keep them from withdrawing into their own world.

Make sure activities include physical activity, small group activities and also large group activities. You want the patient to enjoy both social activities and solitary activities so she gets a range without being overwhelmed.

Three: Provide Stimulation

While activities are a form of stimulation, you should take the time to make sure that your loved one has other types of stimulation. Decorate in colourful and inviting tones and also make sure there is access to the outdoors.

In addition, provide things such as television, radios or other stimuli so your patient is able to watch, listen and do various things even when she is in her own room. Stimulation allows the patient to remain in the present.

Four: Be clear on what you are doing

One thing that many caregivers forget during the day-to-day, is to let the patient know what is happening. By forgetting, you could leave your loved one confused and scared, so make sure you let her know what is happening.

For example, if you have a social activity at the senior center, let her know that she is getting ready for that activity. When you go to the car, tell her she is going to the car so she can get to the activity. When you are driving, tell her where you are driving and so on. The clearer you are, the safer your patient will feel when she is with you.

Five: Avoid Change

Finally, avoid changing things too often. Remember that your patient is going to want to have things remain fairly consistent. Sudden or extreme change can lead to confusion, disorientation and even fear.

Keep a regular routine and schedule for your patient and make sure that you prepare the patient for any sudden changes to that schedule.

In addition, make sure that you keep the home as familiar as possible. While a new couch may be a much needed addition for you, it can leave your patient in turmoil because of the sudden change.

Remember that all of these tips can be applied to anyone with any type of dementia but they are very important for vascular dementia; where there is a sudden progression of the disease.

Chapter 5. Sundown Dementia

Sundown dementia, or sundowning, isn't an actual dementia in itself. It is actually a syndrome that is seen in many different types of dementia, including Alzheimer's. The reason why I am looking at it separately is because it affects many people with dementia and is actually very common.

1. What is Sundown Dementia?

As I have mentioned, sundown dementia is not a separate kind of dementia. It is a syndrome that occurs in many cases of dementia and is known as sundowning or sundowning syndrome.

So what exactly is it? Well, the nurse in the hospital explained it to me. My grandmother's memory seem to be reasonably good in hospital until approx. 6 pm and after that, she would become worse and worse as the evening would progress. I asked the nurse what the reason for it was. She told me that a lot of dementia patients have it: around the time the sun goes down, dementia patients get worse. Their memory gets worse. Their behaviour gets worse. They start wandering around, not knowing where they are. There is no medical explanation for it but it is a fact. The nurse also explained to me that that is the reason why in care homes and hospitals, they make sure all the dementia patients are bathed, fed and changed into their pyjamas before the sundowning effect kicks in. I found that very interesting as I never heard about sundowning before.

My grandmother was really badly affected by the sundowning syndrome, so much so, that the nurses had to strap her in her bed during the night because otherwise she would wander through the halls and walk into other patient's room. That really was painful to watch; my lovely grandmother strapped into a bed, like a criminal.

As we have covered earlier in this book, people with dementia are often left with feelings of confusion. This leads to frustration and also leads to them being disoriented and restless. Although there is no set time when the symptoms of dementia can strike, sundowning is actually referring to a restlessness that occurs in late afternoon or early evening, hence the name sundown.

With this syndrome, the patient becomes extremely upset. She may begin to demand things and she may also become suspicious of those around her. The ability to concentrate on something is minimized and much of her time is spent being disoriented.

In addition, hallucinations are very common with sundowning syndrome, especially during the night time. Patients that are experiencing sundown dementia are often more impulsive and this impulsiveness can often put them at a greater risk of injury. When it comes to sundown dementia, the actual cause is unknown, however, there are some theories as to why it occurs.

One theory is that sundowning occurs as dementia progresses. The less a patient is able to relate to the here and now, the more likely sundowning will occur. The person becomes frantic as the day progresses and it is in an effort to find a familiar place. By the evening, if no familiar place has been found, the patient becomes confused, upset and nervous because she has no sense of security as the day progresses.

Another theory behind this condition is that sundown dementia may occur do to the lack of sensory stimulation later in the afternoon. Lights are dimmed, noises are reduced and the patient does not have as many clues from outside sources during this time. As the evening progresses, the patient becomes more agitated as it becomes more difficult to express her needs.

Other researchers have come up with a number of reasons why sundown dementia occurs. These reasons are:

- *During shift changes:* For patients in long-term homes, the agitation may coincide with the time of day when there are changes in personnel shifts.

- *During busy times of the day:* This can be during meal times, visitation times or any time during the scheduled day when there is a busy period. The extra activity leads to nervousness and creates the right condition for sundown syndrome.

- *When the patient is tired or stressed:* One theory is that sundown dementia occurs as a result of brain disease. During the day, the patient becomes more restless as she begins to tire and this makes her more difficult to settle.

- *When there are too many activities:* It seems to occur on days when there are excessive daytime activities and sensory stimulation. The patient is overwhelmed and slips into the sundown syndrome.

- *Has been linked to hormones:* Some studies have linked sundown dementia to hormonal fluctuations in sick or ill people. When the hormonal fluctuation occurs, the patient becomes stressed and this leads to increased confusion.

- *Occurs more in patients with Alzheimer's Dementia.*

- *Shifts in the internal clock:* This can be due to a number of factors including daylight savings but generally, sundown symptoms occur frequently when the body's "internal clock," also known as the circadian timing system, is disturbed.

- *Health problems may raise the risk of sundown dementia:* Although it has not been thoroughly examined, some indicators point to heart disease, substance abuse, smoking and diabetes as factors leading to a higher risk of developing sundowning syndrome.

Regardless of the cause, sundowning is very hard on caregivers and also on the patient and it is important to seek the proper help when you are caring for a loved one who experiences sundown syndrome.

Before we move onto the symptoms, however, it is important to note that it is not unusual for people without dementia of any kind to experience sundown dementia. In fact, while it is often associated with Alzheimer's or with other forms of dementia, it can actually be a precursor to the condition. Or rather, sundown dementia is the sign that dementia is a problem in the patient.

Another factor that can come into play with sundown dementia is recovery from surgery. This is more common in the elderly and is also more common after anaesthesia is administered. When sundown dementia occurs due to surgery, the effects of the dementia are usually temporary and generally reversible – going away shortly after full recovery. It is when there is a pattern to the sundown dementia that indicator a long lasting problem.

According to Dr. Peter V. Rabins, who is a professor of psychiatry in the geriatric psychiatry and neuropsychiatry division of Johns Hopkins University School of Medicine, *"When there's a pattern to it, it's important to look for triggers or something in the environment. Is there something in the patient's medication? Are their fewer activities? Is there less staffing? There might be things in the environment that may change or things in the patient: biological changes, sleep-wake cycle, and hormone secretion problems. There may be things that can be done, for example, to increase the stimulation for some people, but for others it might be decreasing it. Does it happen every day, how long does it last, how severe is it?"*

As you can see, there is more to sundown dementia and it is for that reason that you need to understand what is triggering the sundown syndrome in your patient as well as the pattern behind it.

2. Signs, Symptoms and Characteristics of Sundown Dementia

As you know, sundown dementia is a syndrome that occurs in many different manifestations of dementia. The word itself implies sleeplessness, or a state of agitated sleep patterns. The terms "nocturnal delirium" or "sleep disturbance" are frequently used for this inadequately explained mind phenomenon.

According to Dr. Glenn Smith, PhD of the Mayo Clinic: *"The term "sundowning" refers to a state of confusion at the end of the day and into the night. Sundowning isn't a disease, but a symptom that often occurs in people with dementia, such as Alzheimer's disease. The cause isn't known."*

Sundown dementia shares the same symptoms of early stage dementia –memory deficiencies, confusion and disorientation- until sunset-time. When the sun starts setting, in the late afternoon or early evening, sundown dementia acquires its own set of symptoms, which I will go over shortly.

One of the most confounding problems behind sundown dementia is that the symptoms often mimic the symptoms of other forms of dementia. In addition, it is "asymptomatic" during the early stages of the disease and it is commonly confused with Alzheimer's or viewed as a symptom of Alzheimer's and not a condition on its own.

The symptoms of sundown dementia are similar to those of other dementias in the elderly; however, they are usually more pronounced. Symptoms that you may see are:

- Severe mood swings

- Restlessness

- Intense confusion

- Paranoia

- Delusions of being watched

- Hallucinations, both seeing and hearing things that aren't there

- Disorientation

- Insecurity

- Being argumentative and demanding

- Reckless behaviour

Although the symptoms are similar to other cases of dementia, they are usually very severe and occur in the late afternoon and early evening.

3. Caring for Someone with Sundown Dementia

When it comes to caring for someone with sundown dementia or sundowning syndrome, there are a number of things that you can do.

First, sundowning has been successfully treated with some medications, however, this does not work for all patients and they should be administered under strict medical observation. Many times, medical treatment usually consists of antipsychotic chemicals -olanzapine and haloperidol for example- with dosages that are tailored for each individual patient. While it may treat the syndrome, the side effects can be quite severe and lead to other problems for the patient.

Second, some patients who suffer from sundowning syndrome do much better in a long-term care facility. Again, this works for a certain percentage of people and in some patients, it could actually make the syndrome worse.

However, if neither of these methods of treatment are ones that you want to pursue, you can manage the symptoms of sundowning. The most important step that you should take before management of sundowning is to educate yourself. Talk to your physician on what he would recommend and also connect with other caregivers. Many times, the best insight comes from people who have worked through sundown dementia.

When you are managing sundowning, there are a few things that you should do and these are:

- *Figure out the time the patient experiences the syndrome.* As you know, many times sundowning occurs during the evening or into the night. Every patient has a time that sundowning syndrome occurs and you need to figure out what that time is yourself. It could be when people are visiting, when there is a shift change, and when there is a break in the schedule. Make sure you document when you see this shift from normal activity to sundowning activity.

- *Make "trigger" periods calm and safe.* Once you are sure of the times and events that trigger the sundowning symptoms, make the effort to make those times calm and peaceful. There are many different ways you can make things peaceful, from minimizing visitors, providing calming periods just before a transition or shifting your schedule so that it is more balanced.

- *Combat night time restlessness with light.* Although you may not realize it, many times, sundowning occurs because of a shift in the patient's internal clock. The best way to combat this is to expose the patient to bright light in the morning for two or three hours. During winter months, a vitamin D lamp can work wonders on fixing the internal clock and during warmer months, some outside exercise can help to fix the internal clock.

- Avoid stimulants in the afternoon. Even if it doesn't seem like much, one cup of coffee or even a really sugary dessert can be enough stimulant to keep the patient up at night. However, it can cause feelings of restlessness and this will increase the risk of sundowning symptoms, including increased paranoia and anxiety.

- Avoid darkness. While many people are not able to sleep with light, people with sundowning dementia are more likely to experience symptoms in darkness. Keeping some lights on so the patient can see if she wakes up will help prevent a trigger from occurring.

- Work through hallucinations. One of the hardest areas to combat with sundown dementia is when the patient has hallucinations. It can be difficult to bring the person back to reality but it is important to stop what you are doing and help them. Stopping a hallucination can be as easy as walking up to the hallucination and waving your hand through it, however, you will need to find out what works for your patient.

- Keep surroundings familiar. Another way to avoid triggers is to keep surroundings familiar. Do not take the patient on trips. In addition, don't change the surroundings too often or too severely. Remember that often sundowning occurs when the patient is not feeling safe.

- Use relaxation methods. Things such as music, calming noises or speaking in low manners are great ways to calm a patient. If the patient is calm, she is less likely to feel restless or frustrated, both of which are very common with sundown dementia.

- Have a pet in the home. Pets are often very good therapy for people with sundown dementia. They are usually very calming and they give the patient something to focus on when they are feeling upset.

- *Keep the patient hydrated.* Water is very important for overall health but it has the added bonus of preventing tiredness and restlessness.

- *Follow a healthy diet consisting of small frequent meals.* Smaller meals are better for people with sundown dementia for the simple reason that smaller meals settle easier. Large meals, especially in the evening around bedtime, can lead to the patient feeling agitated and restless.

- *Make the earlier part of the day busier.* Always plan your schedule so the majority of activities are done in the early part of the day. Make sure you have quiet periods in the afternoon so the patient can feel rested. The less tired the patient feels the less likely sundowning will occur.

- *Daily exercise both in the morning and evening.* Many times, sundown dementia is triggered by an excess of energy. To help prevent this, plan for short periods of exercise twice a day. This will help curb energy and by keeping it small, you will be able to prevent the patient from becoming overtired.

- *Avoid arguing with the patient.* A common trigger for someone with sundown dementia is to argue with them. When you argue, existing feelings of frustration become worse. It can be difficult but make sure that you try to remain positive and calm.

- *Help the patient feel protected.* This is one of the most important things that you can do when you are managing sundown dementia. Many times, when the symptoms occur it is due to feelings of fearfulness. Doing things, such as orienting the patient to her surroundings, will help her feel safe and will help prevent or minimize the symptoms of sundown dementia.

- *Keep connected with the doctor.* Finally, make sure that you are always in regular contact with the patient's physician. He will help you manage the sundown dementia and will make medication changes as is necessary.

4. Shadowing

Before we move on to other forms of dementia, I wanted to talk about one symptom that is frequently seen in people with dementia. In particular, shadowing is something that you commonly see when a person has sundown dementia, which is why I am discussing it in this chapter.

With shadowing, the person with dementia becomes the "shadow" of the caregiver. They follow them around throughout the day and when they can't physically follow the caregiver, they watch. In fact, many times, shadowing will cause them to seek out the caregiver, even during the night.

Shadowing can actually be a very hard experience for the caregiver. While it may seem like a minor problem, shadowing takes away any privacy that the caregiver has. Simple things, such as going to the washroom or even going to bed at night, can become stressful. On one hand, the patient is struggling with you being out of sight and may become frustrated, confused or even fearful. On the other hand, it can be unnerving to wake up in the middle of the night and find the patient staring at you and watching you.

There is no known cause of shadowing, outside of it being a condition that occurs with dementia. Usually, it begins to occur more frequently when the patient is in the later stages of dementia. In addition, shadowing seems to occur more frequently during the late afternoon, early evening or even at night.

Caring for someone who is shadowing.

Like many of the symptoms of dementia, there are ways that you can care for and manage a patient who is shadowing. The very first thing that you should do, is find ways to have your own privacy. Put locks on bedroom doors; put child safety covers on the door handles and so on.

In addition, give the patient a timer or some other way to track time and clearly let her know that you will be gone until the timer goes off. This will help ease her mind and will keep her from trying to find you.

After you have met your needs as a caregiver, there are a few things that you can do to help minimize shadowing in your patient. These are:

- *Distract the patient with activities.* Choose a number of repetitive activities that the patient can do when you are busy. They should be simple to do so they do not frustrate the patient but difficult enough so they do not become bored. Things such as folding clothes or dusting a room can work very well as an activity.

- *Do things when the patient is resting.* Try to find periods of the day when the patient is resting or napping to do your chores so the patient is less likely to notice that you are not with her.

- *Provide the patient with music.* Music has been proven to have a calming effect on many patients, regardless of the prognosis. Give the patient a pair of headphones and put on some soothing music. The patient will be more focused on the music and will be less likely to shadow.

- *Use a food therapy.* This should only be done if the patient is able to chew and swallow without any difficulty. Give her a piece of gum, a small bowl of sugar or something else that is easy to chew. The food will keep her distracted and less inclined to shadow.

- *Make the evenings quiet time.* During the evenings, take that opportunity to spend time with the patient. While it may not help the shadowing, it will keep them in one spot and they will be less likely to follow you around and possibly get hurt.

Shadowing is not something that can be treated. It is a behaviour that the patient cannot control and caregivers need to find a way to work with and manage it. In addition, caregivers should know that many times the patient is not even aware that they are shadowing.

When asked, the patient will have no recollection of doing it and may become upset about the thought of doing it. Instead of trying to work out the shadowing through conversation, simply ignore the topic and manage it instead.

Chapter 6. Lewy Body Dementia

Lewy Body Dementia is the third form of dementia that we are going to be focusing on in this book. One of the main reasons for this is because Lewy Body Dementia is a very common form of dementia.

In fact, it is estimated that nearly 1.3 million individuals are currently living with Lewy Body Dementia in the United States alone. This means that a large number of families and caregivers are affected by Lewy Body Dementia. In addition to the high numbers of diagnosed individuals, there is also a large number of under diagnosed or undiagnosed patients suffering from Lewy Body Dementia. The main reason for this is because this form of dementia often resembles the symptoms found in Alzheimer's disease and Parkinson's disease.

1. What is Lewy Bodies Dementia?

Lewy Bodies Dementia, or rather Lewy Bodies Disease (LBD) is a condition that refers to lumps of abnormal protein structures known as alpa-synuclein. These structures are found in the brain, and more specifically in the parts of the brain where the impairment has taken place.

The disease itself was discovered by a scientist named Frederich Heinrich Lewy who discovered the abnormal proteins in 1912 when he was studying Alzheimer's disease.

The term Lewy Bodies Dementia or LBD is actually an umbrella term that is used to describe two different diseases. The first is Dementia with Lewy Bodies and the other is Parkinson's Disease dementia. Generally, LBD is very difficult for doctor's to diagnose in patients and usually, it is not until the disease has progressed for several years that an accurate diagnosis can be determined. In addition, it is frequently misdiagnosed and improper management is given, which can make the disease worse.

The cause of LBD is unknown and no specific risk factors have been identified. Cases have appeared among families but there does not seem to be a strong tendency for inheriting the disease. There is continuing research on the disease and there may be some indication that genetics play a role in the development of it. One interesting fact with LBD is that it typically affects older patients and is more prevalent in men than it is in women.

2. Signs, Symptoms and Characteristics of Lewy Bodies Dementia

As I have mentioned, the symptoms of Lewy Bodies Dementia is often overlooked in the early stages of the disease. In addition, since the symptoms closely resemble other forms of dementia, it is commonly misdiagnosed. In fact, many doctors are unsure of what LBD is and have a difficult time diagnosing it.

Like other forms of dementia, Lewy Bodies Dementia follows the same stages of progression. It can affect the cognitive abilities of the patient and will affect memory and behaviours. In addition, it can cause neuromuscular irregularities that mimic the symptoms of Parkinson's disease.

Symptoms that are common with Lewy Bodies Dementia are:

- Impaired motor skills. This impairment mimics the symptoms of early stage Parkinson's Disease.

- Hallucinations. Although they can be audible or sensory, many times the hallucinations are visual and are intense and persistent. One characteristic with LBD is that hallucinations can occur even in the early stages of the disease.

- Rapid Eye Movement Sleep Behavior Disorder. This disorder is when the patient has intense dreaming. She may talk in her sleep, toss around while sleeping and have a very fitful sleep. During the day, the patient is usually drowsy and has difficulty functioning because of the sleep patterns.

- Short-term memory loss

- Disorientation

- Difficulty communicating, primarily through speech

- Cognitive impairment

- Impaired thought processes

- Marked behavioural hesitation

- Slipping back and forth, at times intra-day or from day-to-day, between early stage and more advanced stages of dementia

- Difficulty focusing

- Movement idiosyncrasies known as "extra pyramidal" signs. These might include a walking shuffle, a stooping stance and jerking of some muscle groups.

- Loss of balance

- Lack of facial expression

It is important to realize that the symptoms in the early stages can point in the direction of Parkinson's disease; however, if it is Lewy Bodies Dementia, treatment will make the symptoms worse instead of better.

It is important to understand the differences between other forms of dementias and Lewy Bodies Dementia. The reason for this is it will help the physician when diagnosing and the sooner you have a prognosis, the better the quality of life will be for the patient.

Some things that you should know are:

- Hallucinations are more frequent and pronounced in LBD patients. In addition, the hallucinations occur during the early stages of dementia.

- Alzheimer's-type and Parkinson's-type symptoms appear in LBD usually shortly within each other

- Depression is more prevalent in LBD patients

- In LBD movement problems are spontaneous; the symptoms begin suddenly.

- Shaking and tremors are less pronounced in LBD patients.

- LBD is the only disease that loses both dopamine and the neurotransmitter "acetylcholine"

3. Caring for Someone with Lewy Bodies Dementia

Before we look at some tips in regards to caring for someone with Lewy Bodies Dementia, it is important to note that this is a serious disease. In fact, while patients can live for an extended period with some forms of dementia, Lewy Bodies Dementia advances quickly through the stages.

Studies have shown that patients with LBD have a life expectancy of only five to seven years after the onset of symptoms. It is a prognosis that is very hard for patients and family members to hear, since it also means that the dementia progresses at an alarming rate.

With LBD, there is very little that can be done in the way of treatments. In fact, many treatments tend to make the condition worse instead of controlling it. One of the reasons for this is because Lewy Bodies Dementia is a dementia that is not predictable. Patients can progress through the stages in the same way as other dementias; however, it can also jump around through stages. One day, symptoms will not be present at all and then the next, the patient may not be able to walk or communicate.

An important aspect of managing this disease and caring for a patient with Lewy Bodies dementia is to understand the effects that drugs can have on them. The medication can often cause hallucinations or they can affect balance and mobility. Medications that you should avoid if a patient is diagnosed with Lewy Bodies dementia are:

- Tranquilizers such as Neuroleptic
- Anti-psychotic drugs such as haloperidol (Haldol) or thioridazine (Mellaril)
- Benzodiazepines (Valium, Ativan)
- Anti-histamines

The drug Levodopa may be given to treat the shaking and tremors, despite the fact that it may increase the hallucinations in patients with Lewy Bodies dementia. However, some antidepressants have shown to have a positive effect on treating the disease.
With the overall care of a patient with Lewy Bodies dementia, it is important to use the following tips:

- *Keep the patient hydrated.* Falls are very common for patients with LBD so it is important to make sure that they are drinking plenty of fluids. The fluids will often prevent the falls.

- *Assess senses.* Lewy Bodies Dementia is something that often attacks the senses of the patient so it is important to have their senses assessed on a regular basis. Some medications can be used to strengthen the senses and minimize hallucinations.

- *Keep a routine and schedule.* Patients with Lewy Bodies Dementia do much better when they have a set schedule and can expect the same routine every day.

- *Provide a calm environment, especially at bedtime.* It can be very difficult for a patient with Lewy Bodies Dementia to settle down for the evening, so providing a calm environment will help this. Keep noise to a minimum and try to avoid stimulants such as TV and coffee in the late afternoon, early evening.

- *Make tasks simple.* To help the patient remain focus and be successful at a task, make sure that you keep them simple. Always give direction in small steps.

- *Exercise daily.* Exercise is very beneficial for a patient with LBD so make sure she gets exercise both inside and outside. Never allow her to exercise on her own as she can be at risk of falling.

- *Provide stabilizing equipment through the house.* Be sure to have stabilizing equipment throughout the house for the patient. This will help prevent falls. In addition, you may need to have the patient use a wheelchair or walker for stability.

- *Watch blood pressure.* Lastly, take the time to watch the blood pressure of the patient. It is very common for blood pressure to fluctuate in patients with LBD and this is one of the reasons for falls.

Remember that with LBD, symptoms can be bad on one day and fine the next. It is very important that you take this into consideration when you are asking the patient to do anything.

Chapter 7. Other Manifestations of Dementia

Although the main focus on this book is about three specific forms of dementia – vascular dementia, sundown dementia and lewy bodies dementia – it is important to have some understanding of the different manifestations that can occur.

In this chapter, I will go over some of the more common forms of dementia. Unlike the other sections of this book, I will not discuss managing the dementia or how it is treated.

Still, all of the tips used for caring for a person with dementia can be applied to all forms of dementia. Many of the symptoms of dementia are shared across the manifestations. In addition, dementia tends to progress in much of the same ways so the same type of management can work well with more than one manifestation of dementia.

1. Alzheimer's Disease

Alzheimer's disease, or AD, is one of the most common forms of dementia. It is a neurological disease that is caused by a number of factors including genetics, obesity, poor diet and health and medical conditions such as strokes. In addition, some research has linked AD with academic level; with lower academic success being a precursor to AD.

The disease, like all dementias, is progressive and terminal. There is no known cure for dementia; however, it is commonly managed with medication and other treatments. In fact, AD can be slowed down and this has enabled many suffering from AD to live longer lives in a lucid state.

2. Mixed dementia

Mixed dementia occurs when Alzheimer's disease and another dementia – usually vascular, Lewy bodies or Sundown – occur concurrently. It is commonly believed that mixed dementia is much more prevalent than previously analyzed, particularly with the elderly. In fact, studies have shown that 45% of patients with dementia show signs of both Alzheimer's disease and multi-infarct (vascular) dementia.

As a result of these findings, it has become a common theory that physicians should expect mixed dementia whenever an older patient has both cardiovascular issues as well as AD.

For mixed dementia involving AD and multi-infarct disease, physicians have resorted to suggesting improvements in lifestyle. They also recommend healthy diets for the patient in an effort to lower the risk of cardiovascular issues. There are no medications customized for mixed dementia and they are rarely successful in treating or managing the disease.

3. Parkinson's Disease

Many people are not aware of the fact that Parkinson's Disease is a disease that is classified under the umbrella of dementia. While it affects motor skills such as walking and coordination, Parkinson's can also cause cognitive impairments.

Although Parkinson's occurs in younger adults, it usually affects people who are 50 or older. It is also known to run in families, affecting both men and women. When it occurs, it slowly destroys a brain chemical called "dopamine," which controls muscle movement.

Symptoms of Parkinson's disease include blinking, constipation, drooling, difficulty swallowing, problems with balance and walking, a blank or expressionless face, muscle aches and stiffness, and difficulty making movements. The shaking and tremors occur in the limbs at rest, or when the limbs are extended, and in later stages also in the head, lips, tongue and feet.

Further, a Parkinson's patient is usually stooped and will eventually suffer from anxiety, memory loss, hallucinations, confusion, and depression.

As there is no cure for Parkinson's yet, physicians strive to deal with the symptoms, mostly by increasing the levels of dopamine in the brain. There are several medications in use, but they frequently cause severe side effects including delirium, increased hallucinations, and digestive system issues, including vomiting and diarrhea. As the disease progresses, treatment begins to fail until it does not work at all, in any dosage.

4. Frontotemporal dementia

Frontotemporal dementia, also referred to as frontotemporal lobar degeneration, refers to a convergence of diverse and infrequent disorders that primarily impact the frontal and temporal lobes of the brain — the areas largely associated with personality, behavioral performance and speech.

Portions of these lobes wither, and signs and symptoms fluctuate, depending upon the portion of the brain affected. Some patients with frontotemporal dementia experience striking changes in their disposition and become socially ineffectual, impetuous or emotionally lethargic, while others lose the ability to use and comprehend speech.

Although Frontotemporal dementia is frequently confused with AD, having many of the symptoms of AD, it should be noted that that frontotemporal dementia tends to show early signs in a range of ages. In fact, it can occur in people as young as 40, which is much earlier than AD. The other noteworthy symptom that differs from AD, is that frontotemporal patients display a strong appetite and frequently gain weight fast.

5. Creutzfeldt-Jacob disease

Creutzfeldt-Jakob disease (CJD) is a neurodegenerative condition that is both uncommon and lethal in patients who are afflicted with the disease. It affects one out of every million people in the world, making it one of the rarer forms of dementia.

A variant of CJD came into the limelight when "mad cows" and mad cow disease were discovered as a primal cause of CJD. Diseased proteins were discovered in the brains of dead cattle, which were then passed on to human beings when the contaminated meat was eaten.

A relatively widespread epidemic of mad cow disease happened in the UK in the 80's, and one incident of it took place in the U.S. in 2003. Today, blood donations and transfusions from people who have been to areas where mad cow had occurred are not allowed.

CJD keeps incubating for up to twelve years, but then when it starts showing signs and symptoms, death usually follows shortly thereafter, typically within months.

CJD happens when prion protein that is found in several areas of the brain starts changing into odd shapes.

CJD is the deadliest of the dementias that we are covering in this book. By the time a patient's family becomes aware of it, the patient's remaining lifespan is limited to months rather than years.

Mad cow disease was found in the carcass of a cow in California on April 24, 2012, the fourth such case ever in the U.S., which is an indication of how rare the disease is.

6. *Normal Pressure Hydrocephalus*

Hydrocephalus means "water on the brain"; Normal Pressure Hydrocephalus, or NPH, refers to an accumulation of excess fluid inside the skull, leading to swelling and malfunctions of the brain. This occurs frequently for no identifiable reasons.

It can also happen when cerebrospinal fluid (CSF) stops flowing out of the brain. The ventricles of the brain that are filled cannot absorb the additional fluid in their present shape, so they enlarge and put pressure in any viable direction, causing brain damage and destruction.

Many manifestations of NPH resemble general dementia symptoms, such as mood issues, forgetfulness, short concentration spans, confusions, and depression. NPH-specific symptoms consist primarily of what are known as "drop attacks". In these attacks, the patient will suddenly fall, while fully conscious and without having heart problems.

Other symptoms typical of NPH include feet frequently held wide apart, peculiar walking styles, and "gait apraxia," which is difficulty when changes in walking styles occur, difficulty when initiating or preparing to walk, and instability.

7. Huntington's disease

Like CJD, Huntington's disease is a hereditary, "killer" syndrome that has so far proven to be relatively fast acting and incurable. When the composition of genes that are passed from one generation to the next is altered, nerve cells are impaired, with the result that certain brain parts are caused to degenerate.

In addition to typical symptoms of dementia, a patient with Huntington's would have trouble speaking, understanding, thinking, walking, and she would in time become totally dependent on her caregivers for functioning at any level.

Huntington's disease requires upmost resilience on the part of the family and other caregivers, as it progresses quickly. The disease causes twitching and involuntary movements, difficult problems with falls, balance and coordination, and cognitive deficiencies similar to other dementias.

All people who inherit Huntington's disease in time acquire the disorder, and one out of two people who have a parent with Huntington's will acquire it. Only 1-3% of patients with Huntington's acquire it from sources not related to heredity.

It is estimated that in 2009 there were 6000 cases of Huntington's in the UK, and some 30,000 cases in the U.S. making it a rare disorder.

8. Wernicke-Korsakoff syndrome

Wernicke-Korsakoff syndrome is an acute memory disorder usually linked to chronic extreme alcohol abuse, although the direct root is a deficiency in the B vitamin 'thiamin''. It is often included under alcohol-related persisting amnesic maladies.

It carries the names of the German and Russian scientists who, years apart in the late 19th century, described the relation of alcohol abuse to malnutrition, thiamin deficits, sleeplessness, and related failures of the brain. The disease is mostly linked with alcohol abuse, but it can also be a by-product of AIDS, and metastasized cancers.

Symptoms include disorientation, confusion, gaps in memory, problems with learning new information, and "confabulating", or making things up; an activity in which they in fact believe the made-up stories. In addition, motor skills lack steadiness and harmonization.

Physicians can treat the disorder to some extent with high doses of thiamine, but only when alcohol abuse is stopped. In later stages, however, the damage is too severe to be treated.

9. Mild Cognitive Impairment (MCI)

This is also referred to as Incipient Dementia, or "amnesic dementia." It is a relatively benign form of dementia as compared to all the dementias so far described. When a patient has MCI, she is typically in transition between old age and AD or one of the other forms of dementia. Her memory loss is not severe enough to impair her daily functioning. She may need a little help occasionally but many patients with MCI are able to function independently and may remain in this condition for several years.

Chapter 8. Diabetes and Dementia

Before we move on to how dementia affects a patient, it is important to look at a cause of dementia that has become apparent after several studies have confirmed it's link.

To begin, diabetes is a disease where the body is unable to make enough insulin, which is a hormone used to control glucose, or sugar, levels in the blood. Diabetes can occur for several reasons and there are several types where the body either doesn't have enough insulin or cannot use the insulin produced in the body.

For the most part, diabetes has two different types that are the most common. These are type one and type two. There is a third type of diabetes but it is temporary and only occurs during pregnancy, although it does raise the risk of developing type 2 diabetes later in life.

When we are looking at diabetes and how it corresponds to dementia, we are actually looking at type 2 diabetes. This is a diabetes that occurs later in life and is usually a direct result of poor health or genetic predisposition. Some of the reasons why people develop type 2 diabetes are:

- Obesity

- High Blood Pressure

- High Cholesterol

- Impaired Blood Vessels

- Heart Disease

- Circulation Problems

Coincidentally, some of these conditions also increase the likelihood of developing dementia, particularly Alzheimer's disease and vascular dementia. The reason for this is because these types of dementia are often caused by cardiovascular problems.

Another correlation between both dementia and diabetes is that some forms of dementia have many of the same progression. Studies have shown that in some dementia patients, glucose is not used by the brain at all or it is not used properly. This leads to nerve death occurring in the brain. The lack of glucose in the brain leads to a reduced amount of oxygen present in the brain and prevents the brain from communicating.

Finally, beta amyloidal plaques, which are present in the brain of some dementia patients, particularly those with Alzheimer's disease, block the production of insulin. All of these factors prove that there is a very strong link between dementia and diabetes.

With that being said, however, it is important not to panic. While studies have linked those two illnesses together, developing type 2 diabetes does not mean that you will develop dementia. In fact, there is still a lot of information that needs to be found before the link is conclusive.

Yes, there are studies that say there are similarities in the brain of people with some forms of dementia, namely Alzheimer's, and those with diabetes. However, after that point, the similarities are at an end. Diabetes is a dangerous illness on its own and when it is found with dementia, the end result can be catastrophic. Not only does the caregiver need to manage the symptoms of dementia but they also need to manage the symptoms of diabetes.

It is very important to note that a person who is diagnosed with diabetes does not always develop dementia. The main reason to be aware of these studies is so you are aware of the risks involved. Having diabetes will increase the risk of developing dementia.

To reduce these risks, follow these tips:

- Exercise on a daily basis. The more exercise you get, the less likely you will develop diabetes and dementia.

- Eat a balanced diet that is rich in vitamins.

- Take vitamins that are rich in vitamin D and complex B vitamins.

- Be social. Remember that being out with people will help your overall health and well being.

Chapter 9. Behavioural Changes Caused by Dementia

As I have mentioned throughout this book, dementia is associated with a number of symptoms and characteristics. Behavioural changes are one of these characteristics and there are many different behavioural changes that can occur. In fact, often, it is the behavioural changes that cause the greatest shock to family members – a loved one that used to be vibrant and outgoing suddenly becomes withdrawn and aggressive.

Before we go over the different forms of behavioural changes that you will experience, it is important to stress that behavioural changes are completely normal with dementia. In addition, they are very common.

While we may feel that the behavioural changes are deliberate, they are not. Patients with dementia are not able to control many of the impulses that change their behaviour. In addition, family members often bear the brunt of the behavioural change since they are usually the closest to the patient.

When there is a behavioural change, many patients with dementia are not aware of the behaviour and if they are, they are often frightened by it. There is no way for them to stop the behaviour and this can lead to further feelings of anxiety and frustration. When you are dealing with behavioural changes, it is very important to remember these facts.

1. Causes of Behavioural Changes

Although the main cause of a behavioural change is because of the dementia the person has, explaining the cause in that manner is simplifying the problem. The main reason for behavioural changes is often because there are changes taking place in the brain. These changes affect the memory and mood of the patient

71

and can also affect the behaviour. When there are changes in the brain, there are triggers that can set off a behavioural change in the patient. These triggers can be a change in the environment, a shift in health or even a change in the medication the patient is taking.

Another cause for a behavioural change is an underlying psychological problem. While dementia can cause a number of behavioural changes, it is not uncommon for people with dementia to have other problems that are hidden.

If you notice severe behavioural changes in your patient, make sure that you take the time to contact the physician in charge of her care to ensure that there is not an underlying problem.

In this chapter we will go over the different behavioural changes that you may see and at the end, we will offer advice and tips on how to manage behavioural changes in general, as management is often the same for all of the changes.

2. Behaviour: Aggression

One of the most common behavioural changes seen with dementia is aggression. This is often caused by frustration that the patient has due to not being able to remember things or simply because of the confusion that dementia causes in the patient.

With aggression, it can be both physical and verbal. A patient may be verbally abusive, using both abusive tones and abusive language or she may be physically abusive, lashing out with very little provocation.

Aggression occurs for a number of reasons including:

- *Frustration.* This is one of the most common reasons why aggression will manifest. The patient becomes frustrated due to an inability to do something, such as go out due to a locked door.

- *Confusion.* Often paired with frustration, patients that are feeling confused about a situation may lash out aggressively.

- *Fear.* Fear aggression is another area where patients can become aggressive and violent. It is quite common for a patient to lash out when she is scared as a way of protecting herself.

- *Anger.* Anger can manifest in the patient over not getting what she wants. There are other reasons for getting angry when dementia is present and many patients can be violent when they get angry.

- *Lack of stimulation.* While it may not seem like a problem that would cause aggression, lack of stimulation can leave the patient withdraw into her own world. When she is brought out, or because of a hallucination, she can react aggressively.

- *Lack of exercise.* Finally, a lack of exercise can lead to aggression for many of the same reasons that a lack of stimulation can cause aggression.

3. Behaviour: Wandering

Another common behaviour that occurs in patients is wandering. This is where the patient will walk away from her home or familiar surroundings and become lost. It is a very serious behaviour as harm can come to the patient very easily. In addition, the patient can become very scared if they are not sure where they are or even where to go.

When wandering does occur, it is important for preventative measures to be taken. A location tag such as a GPS tracking device or even a safe return bracelet will make it easier to find a patient who has wandered away. In addition, keeping items on them such as snack foods and a small water bottle can keep them safe if they do wander. Another preventative is to have proper locks on doors and to give the patient outdoor pacing time in a secure area so they can wander without feeling restrained.

It is important to note that while medication is frequently prescribed, it often does more harm than good. In fact, medications often make the condition worse and the wandering more frequently. Wandering can't be stopped but it can be moderated enough so that it does not put the patient at risk.

4. Behaviour: Sexual Behaviours

Another common behaviour that can occur with patients who are diagnosed with dementia is sexual behaviours. This could be anything from exhibitionism to a release of sexual inhibitions.

Patients frequently touch themselves in sexual ways and they may also touch others in sexual ways. It is very normal and common; however, it should be addressed.

Like wandering, sexual behaviours are not usually treatable with medication. They need to be properly observed and evaluated to determine when the behaviour occurs and if it is directed towards a specific person. Once it is assessed, steps should be taken to manage the problem such as avoiding the triggers.

5. Behaviour: Screaming

Another behaviour that can be seen, and one that is often very startling, is screaming. Screaming often occurs due to a number of emotions including depression or fear. It can also occur due to an outside trigger such as physical pain or discomfort.

Many times, screaming is often done during care activities – bathing and toileting are common times. Again, there is no medication that can reduce the amount of screaming that is done but there are a few things that should be done. These are rewarding the patient when they are not screaming, ignoring the screaming when you can and using calming methods such as touch or music to prevent and stop screaming.

6. Behaviour: Self-Harming

One form of behaviour that can be detrimental to the health of the patient is self-harming. It is very important for caregivers to be aware of self-harming and to seek help immediately for it.

There is no specific cause for self-harming and it is unclear how frequently it occurs in patients with dementia. Often it is associated with a hallucination or a repetitive behaviour, such as picking at the skin repeatedly. It can be minor self-injury or severe but even the most minor self-harm should not be overlooked.

If you see any self-harm, speak to the patient's physician. Many times, medication can be prescribed to curb self-injurious behaviours.

7. Behaviour: Resistiveness

Resistiveness is a term that is used to describe a patient that is resisting physical care. It can be aggressive but most of the times it is simply a passive resistance. The patient may not help in any way or they may go limp when care is being administered. In other cases, they may lash out to prevent the physical care.

When it comes to caring for a patient with dementia, the resistiveness that is very common in the disorder, is one of the hardest things to work with. It is often one of the main reasons for caregivers to feel overwhelmed and burned out.

While resistiveness is difficult to overcome, many forms of it can be treated with medication, which makes the patient much easier to care for.

8. Behaviour: Hoarding

Hoarding is often a problem that many people experience as an early sign of dementia. It can usually occur at any time during dementia and is simply a behaviour where the patient will begin to gather items and keep them in their home. It could be something as simple as stamps or something like food. The main point of hoarding is that the patient feels there is something missing and will safeguard the items to make sure they are always available.

Hoarding often occurs because of several reasons and these are:

- *Memories of going without.* Memories where the patient did not have certain items, such as food during The Depression, can trigger hoarding. The patient feels the need to always have food near her and she will gather as much as she can. In addition, she will have a difficult time throwing food away, even if it is spoilt.

- *Isolation.* Many times, when a patient feels lonely, isolated or neglected in any way, they may begin to hoard items that help them to avoid those feelings.

- *Being fearful of losing things.* Fear, for whatever reason, can cause a patient to hoard but when they are worried about losing items or being robbed of their items, they are more likely to hoard. In addition, they will often hide their hoarding if they are worried about things being stolen. When they forget where they have hidden them, they react with more fear, believing that the item was actually stolen and this creates a long cycle.

- *Loss.* Loss, not only of cherished items but also of people, can trigger hoarding behaviours. The patient uses items to help overcome the feelings of loss or to take the place of a lost item or person.

Hoarding can be a very difficult behaviour to manage and treat. Often, the items have to be searched out and removed. Treatment needs to be done to help with the underlying emotions behind hoarding and it can be nearly impossible to overcome.

9. Behaviour: Catastrophic Reactions

Catastrophic reactions are often overlooked, but many times, they can be triggered on their own. To explain, a catastrophic reaction is when the patient has a sudden reaction to a trigger. The reaction is not a normal reaction and instead it is reacting to the extreme.

For instance, if there is a minor setback in the day, the patient may begin screaming, throwing accusations at the caregiver and throwing things. Another instance is the patient laughing at a joke but doing so in such an uncontrollable or inappropriate manner that it is extreme.

Catastrophic reactions are very scary and can be overwhelming for both the patient and the caregiver. Many times, it is a catastrophic reaction that is one of the first indicators that something is wrong, before dementia has been diagnosed.

Reactions can be moderated with medication but there are ways to manage the behaviour to keep them from occurring frequently, which we will go over later in this chapter. One thing that is important to remember is that catastrophic reactions are very normal in dementia patients and it is something that you will have to work with as you care for your loved one.

10. Behaviour: Repetitive Actions

The final type of behaviour that you will commonly see in people with dementia is repetitive actions. This is where the patient will do the same action over and over again. Or it could be that they are clingy to the caregiver, also known as shadowing (see the chapter on sundown dementia).

Again, like many types of the behaviours associated with dementia, repetitive actions can be managed with medication, however, it is not always successful.

11. Managing Behavioural Changes

Now that you are aware of the many behavioural changes that you can be faced with, it is important to understand how to manage them. As I have mentioned repeatedly, some behaviours can be managed with medication, however, that won't completely eliminate behaviour.

In fact, many times the behaviours should not be treated with medication and can be compounded if medication is given. One thing that should be mentioned is that management is not the ability to stop the behaviours but it is reduction in the frequency and the severity of the behaviours.

Ways to manage behavioural changes are:

- **Be aware of the triggers.** Before you manage any behavioural change, it is important to watch for the triggers that are causing the behaviour to happen. By understanding what the triggers are you can begin to eliminate the trigger or minimize the effects of the trigger.

- **Remain calm when a behaviour occurs.** Without realizing it, many caregivers reward the behaviour because of their reaction. Remain calm, don't take the behaviour personally and do not raise your voice when you are dealing with the patient.

- **Provide a familiar environment for the patient.** Make sure you avoid making changes in the environment and try to keep it as familiar as possible for the patient. The more stability the patient has, the less likely the patient is to react.

- **Keep a balanced schedule.** Make sure that you have periods of activity and periods for the patient to rest. Some behaviours occur when the patient is feeling under stimulated and others occur when they are feeling over stimulated. Finding a happy balance between the two will help prevent the behaviour changes.

- *Create a calm atmosphere.* Having a calm atmosphere in the patient's home is important as it will prevent many behaviours, especially ones that are triggered by agitation. Make visiting hours as calm as possible and also keep an eye on the patient – removing her from the situation if there is a stressful event. Play music, keep a pet in the home and other calming methods should be utilized as well.

- *Take a step back.* If a behaviour does occur, take a step back and do not touch or restrain the patient as this can often make it worse. Instead, watch the patient to ensure that she does not injure herself and find ways to calm her that doesn't involve touch.

- *Avoid punishing the patient.* It is important to let the behaviour go when the patient has calmed down. Do not hold a grudge and do not punish the patient. Remember that many times a patient with dementia is not even aware that she has had a behaviour change.

Remember to discuss options for dealing with the behaviour and managing it with your patient's physician.

Chapter 10. Medical Problems Associated with Dementia

Before you read this section on medical problems that are often associated with dementia, it is important to read the stages of dementia as well as each individual form of dementia. In each of the chapters, I have gone over medical problems that can occur as well as other obstacles that both caregivers and the patient can experience.

With that in mind, I am going to discuss a number of medical problems that can occur in nearly all cases of dementia, regardless of the manifestation. Again, I will go over the symptoms and believed causes of each medical problem and at the end of the chapter, I will go over ways to help manage these problems.

Remember that dementia is a progressive disease and while it may be easy to manage a problem during the early stages of dementia, as the patient progresses it will become much harder. In addition, the medical problems will become more pronounced as the dementia progresses.

1. Causes of Medical Problems

In general, the main cause of medical problems is the dementia itself. There are a number of psychological problems and even health problems that can arise from the breakdown of the brain cells. As I have mentioned in previous chapters, dementia slowly kills the brain cells of patients.

It is important to note, however, that some of the medical problems that can occur can be both a side effect of dementia or it could indicate underlying medical conditions. It is important to always speak with the patient's doctor whenever a new symptom or medical problem has occurred.

In addition to problems caused directly by the dementia, there are also a number of problems that can be caused indirectly. For instance, a patient may become forgetful about her daily routines and may begin to forget to eat or meet her other needs. Being forgetful in this manner will lead to health problems such as low blood sugar.

2. Medical Problem: Psychosis

Psychosis is a term that refers to psychological problems that can occur for a number of reasons. It is important to note that a high ratio of patients suffering from dementia will experience a psychosis of one form or another; however, psychosis is a condition that can occur without dementia.

With dementia, there are several different ways for psychosis to manifest. These are:

- *Hallucinations:* Hallucinations are very common, especially in sundown dementia. In addition, studies have shown that the occurrence of hallucinations increase for every year that a patient is living with dementia. During the first year, the chance of a hallucination is around 20.1%, the second year it is 36.15%, the third year it is 49.55%, and the fourth year sees the change of frequent hallucinations rise to 51.3%. With hallucinations, visual are usually more common than auditory or a combination of visual and auditory hallucinations.

- *Paranoia:* Paranoia is another way that psychosis can manifest itself when a patient has dementia. Many times the paranoia is tied in with their hallucinations but they may become suspicious of their caregivers. Generally, paranoia is seen more prominently during the middle stages of dementia but it can be seen in the earlier or later stages as well. With paranoia, the patient may believe that people are stealing from her or even that people are trying to kill her.

Psychosis can be very serious and it is often treated with medication. It is important to make sure that the psychosis is diagnosed by a physician as there may be an underlying cause of the psychosis. Generally, though, psychosis is very common in all cases of dementia.

3. Medical Problem: Sleep Disturbances

While many people do not view sleep disturbances as a medical problem, they are actually quite a serious one. Sleep disturbances can hinder your day-to-day life and will affect your overall health. In patients with dementia, this sleep disturbance can compound the problems that dementia present.

One thing that should be understood is that sleep disturbances can be very common as we age. It has been proven that there is often an increase in night time wakefulness as we age. In addition, there is also an increase in napping during the day. However, with dementia, these normal changes are exaggerated and you often see a great increase in night time activity.

With the disruptions in night time sleep cycles, the health, behavioural and emotional problems that are seen with dementia are often magnified. Sleep becomes harder to enjoy for the patient and even naps during the day become difficult. The patient can become withdrawn and will have lower energy levels during the day.

This lack of sleep can leave the patient frail. This fragility will lead to a lack of physical exertion and that will result in even more sleep disturbances. Causes of sleep disruptions due to dementia can be:

- *Nervousness:* If the patient is nervous in any way before she goes to sleep, she may have a harder time sleeping.

- *Depression:* This is very common; patients who are depressed will often have a harder time sleeping during the night. For more information on depression and dementia, read the next chapter on mood changes.

- *Sundown Syndrome:* This syndrome often leads the patients to become agitated during the evening and night time hours, interrupting their sleep patterns.

- *Shadowing:* Another behaviour that is common in dementia patients is shadowing. Shadowing can keep patients awake at night since they are trying to follow, or shadow, their caregivers.

- *Sleep Apnoea:* Sleep apnoea is another reason for problems with sleep and seems to occur with greater frequency in patients with dementia.

With any case of sleep disturbance, it is important to seek the help of a professional. Some medications can be administered to help with sleep but it is important to make sure it does not compound other problems that occur in conjunction to dementia.

In addition to medication, many treatments of sleep disturbances also includes counselling and relaxation sessions so the patient can begin to relax during the night.

Doctors may also recommend the use of bright light therapy, which was discussed in the chapter on Sundown Dementia, as well as increasing exercise during the day. There are ways to help with sleep disturbances but it is important to have it assessed and solved on a patient to physician basis.

4. Medical Problem: Jerking Movements

Another medical problem that seems to affect a high number of patients is jerky or jerking movements. It is important to note that these movements are not repetitive movements or even a fit.

Instead, it is just one jerking movement before the patient comes to rest.

For instance, the patient may kick her leg up just once or her arm may suddenly fling outwards. It is a movement that is completely uncontrollable and many times, the patient is not even aware that it has occurred.

Like many of the problems that you can see, there is nothing that can really be done for it. The main point with this problem is to simply ignore it. Do not restrain the patient or reprimand them for the movement in any way as this can lead to confusion, fear and even aggression.

If the movements seem to become more frequent, speak to the patient's physician.

5. Medical Problem: Constipation

One common medical problem that may occur in patients with dementia is constipation. This often occurs simply because the patient does not properly care for her needs and it is shifted to a caregiver.

The caregiver may give the proper diet and care, however, bowel movements can be difficult to encourage since they are usually under the control of the patient.

When constipation does occur, it can lead to a loss of appetite, which only leads to a deterioration of health. In addition, the patient may experience pain from the constipation but will have difficulty explaining what is wrong to her caregivers.

Usually, constipation can be treated by giving the patient a laxative; however, this should only be done in extreme cases. If it is given too often, the laxative can either aggravate the problem or cause incontinence.

The best way to treat constipation is to follow a proper diet and to encourage your patient to drink water. In addition, proper exercise can help prevent and treat constipation. If the patient has constipation on a regular basis, consult her physician for alternate treatments.

6. Medical Problem: Agnosia

Vision problems are very common in people with dementia and many times it has nothing to do with the diagnosis. In fact, vision problems are common in the elderly and in every age group. With dementia patients, however, when a vision problem is present, the patient may not be aware of it. This can lead them to falling, bumping into things or other behaviours that could harm them.

Another vision problem that seems to be very common in patients with dementia is agnosia. This is a condition where the eyes can actual see perfectly and have no or very little vision loss. However, the brain itself does not interpret the information the eyes are sending. So the patient sees things differently, leading to confusion and paranoia, or the brain may interpret the signal in the same way as normal vision loss.

Many times, the patient with dementia is unable to properly communicate what is happening so it is important for the caregiver to watch for signs of vision impairment. It can be managed with proper diagnose and through the use of glasses and other visual aids.

7. Medical Problem: Pressure Sores

Pressure sores often occur during the more advanced stages of dementia when the patient remains in a stationary position for extended periods. A bedsore is a red sore or patch on the patient's skin, which does not disappear after a few hours.

They can be very painful and are usually the result of sitting or lying in the same position for long periods. They usually form on the part of the body that is in contact with the bed. Pressure sores are very painful and they can be even more so for a patient with dementia, since the sores can be scary and confusing.

It is important to try to avoid pressure sores in the patient. Have them get up to exercise on a daily basis. In addition, keep the skin dry and do not allow the patient to sit in anything damp.

If the sores do occur, consult a physician to determine the best type of treatment.

8. Medical Problem: Loss of Mobility

Loss of mobility is an inevitable medical problem that does occur with patients who suffer from dementia. As the dementia progresses into the later stages, it becomes more difficult for the patient to walk. In addition, before that stage, the patient may experience difficulties with coordination and with dexterity. Simple things, such as turning on a light, may be too difficult for the patient to do.

With the case of dementia, mobility is not often hindered by any physical condition but simply because the brain can no long function properly. When this happens, electrical messages sent to the limb are not transmitted or are transmitted improperly. Although we are aware of the problem and the cause, there is very little that can be done to manage it outside of assisting the patient physically.

9. Medical Problem: Poor Dental Health

Another common problem that is seen with dementia is poor dental health. This is caused by the fact that many patients forget whether they have brushed their teeth or not. As dementia progresses, it becomes even more difficult to manipulate the toothbrush properly.

While the dental health problems can differ from patient to patient, many patients with dementia will have sore gums. In addition, their dentures may not fit properly and those who have their own teeth still may develop cavities.

Poor dental health can lead to other problems such as loss of appetite since eating is painful. In addition, it could lead to the patient speaking less, making it difficult to assess what her needs are.

To help prevent poor dental health, the caregiver should make an effort to brush the patient's teeth on a regular basis. This can be challenging but it is an important part of daily care.

10. Medical Problem: Fits

The final medical problem that is commonly seen is fits. These are times when a limb or even the whole body will begin to make rapid and repetitive motions. It is not like an epileptic fit but instead, more like a jerking movement, however, in a repetitive motion.

The fit is caused by a burst of activity in the brain that sends electrical messages out through the body. The fit could be as simple as a jerking arm or as scary as the body becoming rigid and jerking. There are even cases when the fit prevents a patient from breathing.

Fits can be extremely frightening for the patient, as well as for the caregiver, and it is important to avoid restraining the patient. Make sure that she cannot be hurt while she is in a fit but do not restrain the patient physically.

11. Managing Medical Problems

Managing medical problems should only be done under the direction of a physician. Many are treated with medications;

however, others need to be treated with different forms of therapy.

One thing that is certain is that you should try to keep the environment calm for the patient. Frequently, when there is a medical problem, the patient is very agitated or fearful so having an environment that does not feel safe will compound the problems.

Another important thing to remember is to be patient. While the conditions can get worse, it is not under the patient's control. Avoid getting angry or frustrated, as this will only make the problems harder to deal with. Also, remember that some problems cannot be corrected and are simply something that needs to be ignored.

For any of the medical problems, it is very important to seek the advice of your patient's physician and then go from there.

Chapter 11. Mood Changes Caused by Dementia

The final area that we are going to look at, in regards to changes the patient will be going through, is mood changes. These can range from mild to severe and they can occur without any warning.

In addition, as the dementia progresses, the severity of the mood changes will become worse. Many times, it is the mood changes that lead to the higher level of burnout for caregivers since it can be quite draining dealing with the shifting moods.

As with any other obstacle that a patient can face throughout the battle with dementia, mood changes get worse as the disease progresses. While minor frustrations and worry can be normal in the early stages, so can depression and apathy later on. It is important to view each obstacle as it pertains to the individual patient and while I will explain ways to help manage the conditions later on in this chapter, it is important to speak with your physician when the mood changes are severe.

1. Mood Change: Apathy

Apathy is a mood change that is linked with both a behavioural change – aggression and a medical condition – psychosis. It can occur at any stage of dementia and is not something that should be taken lightly.

When apathy does occur, it is very serious. The patient begins to lose interest in life and has feelings of not caring. It is often described as a lack of motivation.

Symptoms of apathy are often feelings of fatigue, a loss of interest in things around the patient and a motor retardation. In severe cases, cognitive abilities become even more impaired,

89

more so then with dementia. The patient can become severely depressed and it can be difficult to bring the patient out of this.

Although some forms of apathy are treated with medication, it is not always treatable. In fact, some forms of apathy can become worse when medication is administered.

The cause is not known but since it is linked to psychosis and aggression, the cause is very likely to do with those conditions.

2. Mood Change: Loneliness

One common mood change that is seen in many, if not all, patients with dementia is loneliness. Dementia can be a lonely disease, as the patient is often pulled into their own world. It is difficult for them to connect with the outside world and it can be difficult for others to connect with them.

Although feelings of loneliness are often associated with other feelings, such as depression, it does not always have to be treated with medication. Instead, it is more important to draw the patient out of her loneliness.

Make sure that you always interact with the patient in a warm and loving manner. In addition, include the patient in conversations and in decisions. Another tip is to give the patient ways to connect to the outside world, even when they are alone. This can be through a radio, television or even a pet. The key is to use management to treat loneliness since you will see the best results by treating it in this manner.

3. Mood Change: Boredom

Another mood change that is common for patients with dementia, especially those in long-term care facilities, is boredom. This is simply a listlessness or even restlessness that occurs because the patient has nothing to do.

Frequently, boredom is not communicated to the caregivers. In fact, it can often be overlooked since the patient is not able to explain what is wrong. Instead, the patient will act out, usually through agitated behaviours or even aggression.

Boredom can be easily treated by giving the patient something to do. This can be as simple as the patient having books to handle and leaf through or more complex, such as a craft like clay shaping.

Whatever you choose to offer the patient, make sure that there is nothing harmful. Small buttons or items that can break should never be given to a patient to help overcome boredom. In addition, all art activities should be supervised.

4. Mood Change: Depression

Depression is both a mood change and a medical condition that you can experience. It is important to always contact the patient's physician if she is experiencing any signs of depression.

It can be caused by a number of physical imbalances and also as a side effect of psychosis. In addition, depression can often be related to the prognosis around dementia.
One thing that should be noted is that depression does not get worse or better as the disease progresses. It can also make some behaviours, such as aggression, worse.
If you suspect depression, it is very important that you contact the patient's physician to make sure that it is treated properly. Many times the treatment for depression is through medication and counselling.

5. Mood Change: Anxiety

The final mood that I wanted to talk about is anxiety, which can include fear, worry and even terror. Anxiety is very common in dementia patients through all stages of the disease. Patients will feel anxious about their lost memories, their inability to function on their own and their deteriorating health.

In addition, patients can be anxious, from perceived situations that can be misunderstood or even a hallucination. While anxiety is a constant mood that has to be monitored, it is important to remember that it can affect both the person's quality of life and her health.

If you do not manage the anxiety properly, the patient's health will quickly deteriorate. The anxiety will also grow until it becomes something that is uncontrollable.

Anxiety has been treated successfully with medication; however, this is not always the best option. Instead, you should try to provide a calm environment for the patient. Another thing that you can do is to bring in a pet or find ways to help the person relax, such as with music. Management is often the best choice for dealing with anxiety but always discuss options with the physician.

6. Managing Mood Changes

Managing a patients mood changes are done in many of the same ways that you would manage behavioural changes. It is a matter of setting up the environment so it enables the patient to have the best outlook.

As I have already mentioned, some mood changes, such as depression, can be treated with medication. It is important to note, however, that not everything can be treated with medication. Some things will need to be managed carefully with therapy while other moods can be managed through following the tips.

- *Be aware of the triggers.* This should be done with any type of reaction, whether it is a mood or a behaviour. Stress, overexcitement, not enough stimulation and even feeling unwell can lead to a mood change so make sure you are aware of the trigger.

- *Provide a calm environment.* Dementia patients cope much better in environments that are calm and warm. An environment that is too busy can cause frustration or stress and this can lead to many mood changes. Try to stick to a schedule and avoid a busy environment.

- *Provide a familiar environment for the patient.* This is important in all aspects of managing dementia but it is important to make sure that you avoid making changes in the environment. Try to keep it as familiar as possible for the patient. The more stability the patient has, the less likely the patient is to react.

- *Avoid getting the patient to explain her mood.* Although some dementia patients can explain what is wrong, many cannot. Asking them to explain a mood will only cause the patient to become stressed and lead to other problems.

- *Keep the patient busy.* Another important way to manage some moods is to keep the patient busy. Have activities for the patient to do and also make sure that there are social activities arranged. Dementia can make patients feel isolated so get them out and away from that isolation.

- *Allow periods to relax.* Finally, when you are creating a busy schedule, don't fill it too much. Everyone needs down time to relax and if you make it too busy, you can cause the patient to feel a high level of stress and anxiety.

Again, it is important to contact your patient's physician to help you manage mood shifts and changes.

Chapter 12. Case Studies of Dementia

Now that we have gone over the many different types of dementia that can occur, I wanted to look at some case studies before we move into the actual caring of a patient. These case studies will help shed some light on how dementia affects families and will also show you some of the choices that caregivers have to make.

1. Case Study Number One: Amy's Mum

Amy was a woman who had a busy life. She worked at a government agency in the United States as an inspector and during the rest of the time; she cared for her mum who was suffering from the early stages of dementia. Amy's mum had developed many of the symptoms of Sundown Dementia but through some effort, Amy was able to keep her mum at home with her.

Amy learned early on during the care that she needed a support network to help her with her mum's care. She began by enlisting the help of a neighbour, who pitched in with the chores and making sure Amy's mom was safe and secure while Amy was working. She also had an in-home nursing service come in and help with the demands that caring for her mum presented.

When Amy was home with her mum, she was a devoted and knowledgeable caregiver and was constantly updating her knowledge on how to deal with the dementia her mum had.

Amy had learned early on that a good nutritional diet, as well as exercise and keeping the mind busy in a positive manner, delayed, and many times reversed, the progression of her mum's syndrome.

For that reason, there was always a cooked meal for dinner at her home, and she took her mum out on walks every day right after an early dinner. She kept walks set to the times when there was still some sunlight to help prevent any confusion or fear from occurring.

Typical of other patients with early-stage dementia, Amy's mum was often aware of her short-term memory loss. This contributed to feelings of inadequacy and frustration, which also contribute to depression. This depression and frustration can prove challenging for both those living with Sundown Dementia as well as for their caregivers.

Amy combated that ferociously, reading to her mum, asking her mum to recount events and stories from the past, and encouraging her mum to do as much as possible for herself, even if Amy ended up do it again the right way.

When they watched a little bit of television, Amy would ask her mum to tell her what was going on, and what she thought would happen next. If someone were singing, Amy would start singing along, which encouraged her mum to join in.
It was through these many different techniques that Amy tried to slow the progress of her mum's sundown syndrome. However, many of the things that Amy did had a slowing effect only and the disease continued to progress.

a) *How the difficulties increase as the disease progresses*

With each progression of the disease, Amy began to find more problems arising. It became increasingly hard for Amy to manage the dementia and her mum began to develop an indifference to the care she was receiving. As it continued to progress further, Amy's mum became unable to care for herself properly and began to rely heavily on the care that Amy and her support team gave her.

In addition to the added stress of the progressing dementia, parts of Amy's support network began to deteriorate. The neighbour, who usually cared for her mum during the day, became more hesitant to provide care. Amy's mum would usually start her day in a positive manner but as the day progressed, her mood would shift drastically. By sunset, Amy's mum would be agitated and aggressive, something that the neighbour was not prepared to deal with.

When Amy arrived home from work, she would be faced with a mum who was already slipping into the symptoms of Sundowning and it would become a difficult night while she tried to calm her mum enough to get some sleep.

As this continued to go on, Amy's mum began to become confused about the people in her world. She frequently forgot who Amy was and during those times, she would become combative. She would refuse to help with simple tasks and would refuse to help with her own care.

Amy's mum had lost the ability to concentrate and started showing signs of anger emanating from her frustration. All the memories that Amy had of a mum who had taught high school math for 30 years were gone. The outgoing, vivacious woman that had loved to travel and spend time with family was disappearing. As each part of her mum seemed to be erased beneath the onslaught of dementia, Amy found it harder and harder to provide the proper amount of care.

In addition to the confusion during the day, Amy's mum also began waking up two or three times at night – many of the times panicked and totally confused. To combat this problem, Amy left the whole floor where they slept fully lit at night and removed all obstructions to prevent accidents. During the night, she would have to continually wake herself up to find her mum, who often got up and wandered around the house, and take her back to her bed.

As time progressed, there was almost a daily change to the living patterns that Amy's mum experienced. Every new symptom led to new challenges that had to be overcome. Then, one of the worst moments of Amy's care giving experience occurred when her mum became incontinent.

b) Challenges of Deciding on Extended Care

Up until that point, Amy had been proud of enabling her mum to live independently at home. When faced with incontinence, Amy had a desperate choice to make – either get a caregiver during the day or start looking for alternate living arrangements for her mum.

The choice wasn't that easy to make. On one hand, the assisted living facilities that could provide the proper care for patients with dementia had a very high price tag. A minimum cost was roughly $45,000USD per year. For places that provided better treatment and private rooms, the costs were close to double.

On the other hand, caregivers, especially those that were required for long hours, also cost a large amount and it was difficult to find a caregiver who had the proper experience with dementia.

Amy could not afford the long-term health facility; neither could she afford to stop working to take care of her mum full time. The neighbour had stopped caring for Amy's mum during the day and many of the other support networks that she had in place were proving to be inadequate. Finally, after some searching, Amy was able to hire a caregiver to care for her mum 5 days a week while she was at work. While the caregiver did have some experience dealing with dementia, she was not as equipped as Amy would have preferred but it was still a relief to know that her mum was in good hands while she was working.

While Amy was trying to establish the proper care, her mum's dementia was progressing rapidly and was quickly destroying the nerve cells in her brain.

Some days, Amy's mum was more coherent than on other days, however, her ability to communicate her needs and to also care for herself was in constant decline. It was this rapid decline that caused a high level of apprehension in Amy.

For primary caregivers, like Amy, the changes to someone living with Sundown dementia can be dramatic. She had to take time off several times and she had to frequently interview several caregivers to help her with her mum. One thing that was evident was that not every caregiver was suitable to care for someone with Sundown Dementia.

A caregiver has have patience, and be compassionate under all circumstances, with the emphasis on *all*.

Like patients with Alzheimer's, a patient with sundowning is capable of combativeness and aggression that can be overwhelming to a caregiver that is not aware of this problem. Amy was aware of that and she went through several caregivers, as it was impossible to foresee what her mum's temperament was going to be on any given day.

As the search was sapping the strength from Amy, her mum was losing whatever energy she had left in her and was becoming apathetic. In the middle of the night, she would wake up and fight with the hallucinations that seemed to plague her on a nearly constant basis. Hardly a night would pass by when Amy could get a decent night's sleep.

Despite all the effort that Amy put out, she experienced a high turnover rate for her caregivers. Every time she lost a caregiver, she would lose more time at work and would have to go through the gruelling process of trying to find another caregiver. Her world was slipping away as surely as her mum's reality was

.

c) Deciding on Assisted Living Facilities (ALFs)

In the end, with remorse eating away at her, Amy made the decision to find an assisted living facility for her mum.

As with other assisted living facilities, the facility where Amy placed her Mom offered activities. An activities person would encourage all who wanted, and were able, to join her in a large living room. There the activities person would make the patients do exercises with small weights for those who could, encouraging and coaxing the patients as they did the routines. For Amy's mum; however, exercises and socializing was out of the question.

She had reacted to the new dwellings in a heart-wrenching manner. The unfamiliarity, the new caregivers and the new schedules overwhelmed her and it appeared as though Amy would have to bring her back home for her mum's own safety.

At first, Amy spent all of her time in the facility. She missed work and would sleep on the couch so she could be near her mum. During the daytime, her mum withdrew into her own world but at night, that world would become a frightening reality and she suffered from severe hallucinations. In fact, during the first week, she slept less than two hours. At the end of the week, Amy had to return to work but she spent much of the time worrying about her mum.

It seemed as though her mum was losing the battle with sundown dementia. She lost roughly 8 pounds that first week and she became unable to move. She was aggressive during the evenings and the facility began to discuss options such as restraining Amy's mum, which would have made things worse.

However, after several agonizing weeks, her mum found a compass in the facility and began to find some peace. This was due to a compassionate aide who Amy's mum had taken a liking to. Finally, much to Amy's relief, her mum had the care she needed and was doing much better than she had in years.

d) How sundowning can tear the family apart

However, the same could not be said for Amy. Over the years, she had developed the habit of spending all her free time with her mum. When she didn't need to as much, she found it difficult to function and would still go to the facility to be with her mum instead of dealing with her own problems.

Her savings were being depleted from the costs of the in-home caregivers, the assisted living facility itself and also from the cost of having a private duty staff in the facility. The costs were mounting up and she found herself struggling with the burden of debt and also with the burden of guilt for having her mum in a facility with people who didn't love her.

In the end, Amy was left with the decision, to take care of her mum completely, at great expense to herself or to find alternative ways. She was letting her own health fall to the wayside and if she continued in that manner, it wouldn't be long before she too was faced with the prognosis of dementia.

After a heart-wrenching journey, Amy finally made the decision, through the help of some professionals such as her mum's business partner, to move her mum to a Medicaid-certified nursing home. The help that she needed was there and Amy was able to spend the last few years with her mum while still being able to care for her own needs.

2. Case Study Number Two: My Grandmother

I have already touched on the story of my grandmother in the foreword but it is an important case study that has affected much of the information I have provided in this book. While I have been a part of the many different choices that were made on behalf of my grandmother, this case study is one that is still developing and while we have had many successes, we know that it is only a matter of time before her dementia will progress further.

To begin, my grandmother has always been an intelligent, active and fit woman. Even at the age of 86, she lived independently in Belgium. She spent her time travelling; going on holiday, going to the theatre, restaurants and visiting her friends. She was enjoying her life fully and had no financial worries as she was lucky that my grandfather had provided for her after he died.

Even her health did not worry her; except for an irregular heartbeat that she had for 30 years, her health was exceptional. However, as she grew older, the irregular heartbeats became more frequent and her primary physician sent her to a heart specialist.

The heart specialist, in an attempt to investigate the reason behind her irregular heartbeats, ordered a series of injections that would enable him to run a number of tests. The injections were standard and they were administered underneath her skin, around her stomach area.

So without much worry from my grandmother or anyone in the family, she scheduled the appointment for a Tuesday morning in December of 2011. The nurse arrived promptly on time and after the minor prep, began the first series of injections. Everything seemed to have gone well as far as anyone knew. Mum phoned my grandmother every day to see how she was but on the fourth day after the injections, it was immediately clear within seconds of my grandmother picking up the phone that something was wrong. My mum could hear it in my grandmother's voice. My mom instantly phoned her brother and told him to go and see my grandmother. On his arrival, he called for an ambulance and my grandmother was rushed to hospital. My mum immediately dropped everything she was doing and started her journey to Belgium.

At that point, no one was sure what was going on. All we knew is that the normally vibrant 86 years old was no longer vibrant. She was limp and had lost a lot of energy. The diagnosis at the hospital was bad. She had a hematoma, which is a localized collection of blood outside the blood vessels, under her stomach skin at the site of the injections. The hematoma was 8 inches (19cm) long and was 5 inches (11cm) deep.

It was a serious condition. My grandmother's body was trying to cope with the hematoma by using up the sugar reserves that she had in her body. At this stage, her sugar level so low that she close to slipping into a coma. It was continuing to use the sugar reserves and her body was deteriorating rapidly.

It was clear that the hematoma was caused by the injections but further testing was needed to determine why a usually safe procedure had those side effects. In the end, it turned out that either my grandmother had an allergic reaction to the injection or her liver was unable to cope with the infections. Through further tests, it was determined that her liver was in poor health and the injection should never be given to a person with a bad liver.

One thing was certain, we would never know if the hematoma was caused by the medical staff or if she had simply been "really, really unlucky." Her doctors wanted us to believe the latter.

Regardless of the reason, we were left with a grandmother that had a life threatening hematoma. From the size of it alone, blood circulation to her brain had been extensively reduced and at times even stopped. In addition to this problem, she had developed both a urine infection and a lung infection.

She spent 10 days in the hospital before she was released, however, within 5 days after being released, her health deteriorated again and she was back. The hematoma was a problem that would take at least 6 months to disappear and her blood sugar levels continued to be a problem, which was the reason for the second trip, by ambulance, to the hospital.

Due to the low blood sugar levels and the oxygen not flowing to her brains properly (due to the hematoma), irrevocable damage had been done to her brain but at the time, we were unable to determine exactly how much damage was done.

One thing that it did teach us is that you don't always have advanced notice that something this life altering is going to happen. Many times, you have a stable family life when, suddenly, dementia thunders in whether you are ready or not. It does not consider whether you have made the necessary preparations or not or even if you know what to do next.

During my grandmother's stay in the hospital, she suffered from really bad from sundown dementia. Through most of the day she was completely normal without any cognitive problems. However, at 6 p.m. she transformed and didn't know anything, not even how old her eldest child was (she had 5 children).

Periodically during this time, she also became incontinent. She had been a proud woman, self-sustained and completely independent, and now she had to accept the adult under-pads she had to wear. This was truly disheartening for her and for everyone in the family –watching her go from a very active, healthy woman to a woman that could not attend to her most basic needs in a matter of weeks.

My mum had to spend months and months in Belgium, leaving my own family in the UK to prove people wrong. You see, everybody said she should go to a home for the elderly but the problem was that grandmother absolutely hated that idea. My mum wanted to do what my grandmother wanted and what we all knew was best for her.

Effort was made and in doing so, the world was turned upside down in an effort to get her back into her own home where she wanted to be. At every turn, those involved in her care were challenging the choices of my mum and the rest of the family. But after months of working towards the goal, my grandmother is finally living on her own in the home she has loved for years.

In addition to the struggle of getting her back into her home, we found ourselves faced with a loss of friends. People who had known my grandmother for decades were suddenly not there for her. Close friends, best friends and even the ones who my grandmother had gone above and beyond for.

One example of this was when we found out my grandmother's best friend no longer wanted to go on holiday with her. The reason was simply because my grandmother "was not the person she used to be" and she did not want to take the responsibility for her. My mum had to deliver the news that my grandmother can no longer go on holiday with her friends, something she basically lives for... my grandmother was devastated.

Personally, it was very sad that her friend, who she has been friends with for 20 years, doesn't want to look after her, however, we understood that her friend was too scared if something would happen on holiday that it would be her fault.

Despite these hurdles, everyone in the family is quick to say that we were lucky to have the financial resources to accomplish what my mum did. In fact, my mum is the first to admit that she would not have been able to do much of what she would have wanted to accomplish had she not had the means.

However, even with the means, it has definitely not been easy, and I am still very proud of my mum for her accomplishment, for other people might have taken "the easier road travelled" and put her into a care home.

In this book we repeat, in many different ways, that although keeping a patient at home is almost always the best option, people's circumstances don't always allow that.

What was Put in Place for Grandmother.

As you know, my grandmother has experienced a more positive outcome despite the obstacles that she has and continues to face. Many people are unable to provide the necessary means to support a loved one with dementia in their own home. For us, a number of different efforts were made to ensure that this was possible. Some of the things that were done:

- A nurse was hired to go to her house four times per day to give her medication. It is very important that her sugar levels stay where they should be since low sugar levels can lead to more damage to her brain and can also lead to serious infections.

- A nurse comes every morning to wash her and see to her morning hygiene needs.

- Three times per week another caregiver comes to take care of the household chores. Things like tidying the house, shopping, collecting mail and so on.

- There is a day-clock on her table (a clock that tells the day, date and month), as pictured below. The reason why we thought that was a good solution is because when grandmother was looking in a TV magazine to see what was on, she would be looking on the wrong day, not knowing what date it was.

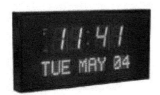

- Once a week she goes to a day care centre for the elderly.

- Her apartment has been re-arranged so she has "walk-space" everywhere.

- There are large pieces of paper throughout the house on stand up boards. These are there so she can remember things. In addition, every door out of the house has a list of things she should take with her when she leaves such as her wallet, keys and cell phone.

- She has a neck-alarm to call for help if she falls and an "I lost my keys" alarm if she loses her keys.

- All glass items have been removed from the home to avoid cuts and other injuries.

- All alcohol has been removed from the home.

- The house has been safety proofed. All "potential" dangers are solved: no curly rugs, no wires hanging around and so on.

- There are cameras set up in the home, which can be accessed from the family member's home computers. This enables us to check if she is okay without interfering with her privacy.

- 2 spoonfuls of coconut oil are administered every day to help improve brain function.

- The stove is turned off to prevent fires as a warm meal was provided for her every day.

- Fire alarms have been installed in every room of the home.

- A rotating schedule is set up with aunts and uncles in the family. Every weekend, one of her kids is responsible to cook her meals and take care of her.

- A schedule has been created so she has something happening every day. This will help prevent her from fading away into her own world and will keep her as grounded in reality as possible.

- She has a GPS system in her shoes that allows family members to know where she is at all times. My mum could see, just by logging into the computer, where her mum was. Very clever equipment.

- We put a paper with all family member's phone numbers in her handbag and again, in her purse.

Although it does seem like a lot of things being done for my grandmother, it is what is needed to ensure that she can stay in her home as long as she wants to. Again, it is through my mum and her siblings that this is possible.

Right now, my grandmother can still do many things that she did before the diagnosis of vascular dementia. She can take the bus to her "regular places" she used to go to because this is an "old" memory, and she can still remember things linked to old memories.

New memories are where many of the problems are occurring. She cannot cope with anything new, even things that seem simple, such as a new remote for the television. She has lost her short-term memory completely and this makes it very difficult for her. Although my grandmother is in the early stages of dementia, we all know she will only get worse.

Naturally, we have all learned a lot from my grandmother's experience, and the experience remains ongoing as I write these words. There is always a new reason to return to Belgium and take care of issues that have occurred.

One of the early lessons that was learned was in relation to one's health generally and dementia. Grandmother's sugar level or even a mild infection has an immediate and adverse effect on her dementia. We try hard to keep her eating healthy food, drinking lots of fluids, and taking vitamins that are prescribed for her. The nurse told me, that, very often, with dementia patients, every time they get an infection. their conditions gets worse.

Update May 2013:

A few things happened and my mum realised something needed to change as my grandmother got worse.

- We discovered that the meals that were delivered to her daily, were hidden in the wardrobe, so she did not eat them.

- When the nurses were scheduled to come in at a certain time, grandmother would not be there because she said "I don't need a nurse, I am perfectly fine".

- My mum made an appointment with the hairdresser for my grandmother, only to conclude that grandmother was going the wrong way and went to a butcher instead. My mum was following her at the time (without grandmother knowing this), to see if she would find her way home, which she didn't.

- In a restaurant, grandmother would pay the bill and 5 minutes later she would ask to pay the bill again.

- When shopping, grandmother told the cashier, she never had a pin code for her card, why should she have one now? Of course, she forgot her pin number and even forgot that you need a pin number to pay in a shop.

Because of all these incidents, mum decided to have further tests done to see if grandmother could keep on living on her own. She was assessed in a special institution where they did tests to see if she could still live on her own without being a danger to herself or to others.

The conclusion was that unfortunately she wasn't able to do that because during the tests, she left the iron on, when instructed to switch it off after use and she left the cooker on after cooking and put some newspapers on top of the cooker.

My grandmother now has a full time carer, living in with her, 24/7. My mum (after a long search) found a company that provides that service. If you are living in Belgium or Holland, here are the details of that company : www.seniorcare24.be . Perhaps Seniorcare24 knows companies in other countries that can help you, just contact them.
Grandmother is now very happy with her full time carer and we, as a family, feel good as we know she is being looked after very well.
She can still enjoy her life, as she wishes to enjoy it. She can go where she wants to, when she wants to but the carer goes with her, everywhere she goes.

Grandmother is happy, mum is happy, I am happy, all other family members are happy!

If you can afford it, from everything that I've seen in the dementia world, the option of letting the patient live in their own home, in familiar surroundings is always the best option. I can now see how happy my grandmother is. Without my mum disagreeing with other family members and with doctors, grandmother would probably be in a care home now.
You see, you don't always have to believe what the doctors or nurses say is best for the patient. Go with your gut-instinct with what YOU think is best as YOU know your patient best, not the medical staff. Of course, always take their opinions into account, whatever you decide.

The main reason why mum insisted that grandmother needed to stay at home as long as possible is because, when grandmother was still very well, she told mum that, if anything would happen to her, she would prefer to stay in her own home. So my mum did what grandmother wanted, even if it was very often difficult for my mum as she needed to turn her life upside down, before we had the solution of 24/7 live in car

Chapter 13. When Additional Care is Needed

Anyone who has ever been faced with that tragic event that confirms that a loved one has dementia, is faced with the decision on whether or not it is time to provide care for their loved one.

The biggest problem, however, is deciding when to make the choice about additional care and also how to move forward with the care.

1. Where to keep your Patient

If your patient has a home and family close by, and if family circumstances permit it, the first option to examine naturally is the one of keeping your patient in her own home.

If you are considering whether to provide the care yourself or hire a professional caregiver, there are these considerations to take into account:

- If your patient is alert, ambulatory, continent, and does not have an illness that requires her, for example, to need to be seen by registered nurses and physicians all the time, you can be her caregiver yourself. You will need to manage her household, do some housekeeping, buy groceries, take care of all the financials like paying bills, managing money, prepare meals, keep her company and take her out occasionally.

Be warned, it is not easy, the dangers of stress and depression are overwhelming; but if you have to, then you will, hopefully only until you find better and longer-term solutions. In fact, you may have no choice in the matter, at least for a few days.

- If your patient is non-ambulatory, think "transfers": from bed to wheelchair, to couch, back to wheelchair, over the edge of the bathtub, and so on, all day long.

With the patient's dementia, sundowner's or Alzheimer's, she cannot be left unattended; your entire life will depend on keeping her from wandering outdoors, causing herself harm in many ways, or setting the house on fire.

- If your patient is incontinent, you will have to deal with incontinence, and a daily routine that is punctuated by unpleasant incontinence.

If the patient is any of the above three, non-ambulatory, confused, incontinent or, as was mentioned previously, if she has a debilitating illness, then you are going to need to hire a professional caregiver, only until you sort things out. You may hire a professional caregiver for enough days until you place the patient in another setting outside her home, but you will nevertheless have to hire a caregiver.

2. Keeping the patient in her own home

Everybody I spoke to told me that the very best thing is to keep the patient at home for as long as possible. I have seen many examples of people being admitted in a care home and very quickly getting a lot worse. Most patients would function much better in the familiar surroundings of their homes.

Her familiarity with the environment where she lives and has lived over time would play an invaluable role in dragging out the progressive nature of her illness as long as possible and keep at least some of the demons of dementia at bay –could be for several years.

From the affectionate and humane point of view, the same applies. She would follow the routine set for her and her alone, and not for her together with the rest of the residents in an institution. She would not be at the mercy of the rigors and disciplines that institutions have to adopt.

All planning and routines would be customized to her needs. At home is where the best care can be implemented, the best lifestyle, with nutritionally sound meals, exercise, hygiene, and companionship.

What I have just described is also somewhat utopic and fraught with risks.

Financially, this is one of the most expensive of the options, for not only will she need professional help day and night, but there will be the added costs of living: the inability to sell the house, the upkeep of the house, and living expenses for her and her caregivers.

3. Are you going to be her caregiver?

At this point, I would like to introduce you to care giving, not in a clinical sense, but the way I have experienced and researched it myself, and the way it is going to be most useful to you.

It is not easy, the dangers of stress and depression are overwhelming; but if you have to, then you will, hopefully only until you find better and longer-term solutions. In fact, you may have no choice in the matter, at least for the first few days after the initial shock.

If the patient is not alert, if she has short-term memory loss, Alzheimer's, or any of the other forms of dementia, she cannot be left unattended; your entire life will depend on keeping her from wandering outdoors, causing herself harm in many ways, or setting the house on fire.

If the patient is incontinent, you will have to deal with incontinence, and a daily routine that is punctuated by unpleasant incontinence-related tasks, such as occasional diarrhoea.

112

You may hire a professional caregiver for enough days until you place the patient in another setting outside her home, but you will nevertheless have to hire a caregiver.

4. Telling Your Loved One She Needs Help

The last thing that I want to touch on is telling your loved one that she needs help, whether this is through your care or outside care. Generally, letting a person with dementia know that she needs help can be very difficult. If the dementia is still in the early stages, she may have a hard time understanding why you need to take the measures you are. If it is in the later stages, then you will be faced with agitation and fear.

Although I would love to tell you that there is an easy way to broach this subject, there isn't. However, that doesn't mean it should be avoided or you should go and make changes without letting the patient know.

When it comes to telling them, there are actually two different ways that you can do so.

1. Ask the doctor to be there with you and your family to discuss the prognosis and the decision to provide care for the patient. Usually, a doctor has been there for all of the stages of dementia and can offer you and your patient ample advice as you are moving forward.

2. Tell your patient when you are doing something pleasant, such as going out for lunch together. Do it in a small group of only 1 or 2 people to help avoid overwhelming the person.

When you are telling your loved one that they need care, make sure that you do it in this manner.

- Tell them on the day that the changes will be made. While this does seem sudden, telling them on the day of a move or a major change will help prevent a lot of agitation for the patient. Depending on the stage of dementia, this is actually the only way to do it as they may forget if you tell them too early.

- Be patient with them. Having to go from a person who can care for themselves, to a person who is cared for can be very difficult. Expect some agitation but remember that this is normal.

- Let them make some of the minor decisions. While the majority of the decisions will have to be made by you, make sure that you allow them to make some of the minor decisions regarding their extended care, if this is still possible. This is even more important when your patient is in the early stages of dementia.

It is not an easy task but if you tell your patient with patience, love and respect, you are sure to make it a bit easier on everyone involved.

Chapter 14. Providing Care as a Family

When it comes to caring for a loved one with dementia, many families choose to care for that person themselves. After all, it can be costly to hire outside care and many families want their loved one to have a piece of dignity that they find is lacking in nursing homes.

Be open about your budget and your own limitations and don't be afraid to ask for help when you need it.

1. Safety Devices

It is very important to provide a safe home for your patient and this should start with safety devices. There are hundreds of devices on the market that cater to the safety and comforts of an elderly person, including those designed for patients with dementia.

At the end of this book, there is a variety of links to suppliers of elderly safety equipment. Although the cost can be expensive, some suppliers will charge your insurance directly, which will save you costs. It is important to note that some of these supplies are reimbursed by your insurance company.

When my mum implemented safety in my grandmother's home, it reminded me of all the things one would do if you have small children. **So, sadly, in a way, a dementia patient, often is best looked at, from a safety point of view, as if she is a baby/child. Therefore, whatever you would do to protect your baby, do the same for the dementia patient.**

Supplies that you should have for your home are:

- *Bathroom Safety Devices:* You should have horizontal grab bars on at least two sides of the tub, a vertical bar to help the patient get into the tub, bars around the toilet, a high chair for the

115

toilet, shower chair with a back, non slip bath mats,shower stools to sit on, transfer benches and non-slip mats.

- *Mobility Equipment:* Things such as walkers, canes and wheelchairs as needed.

- *Special Bed:* Beds that have sides on them to prevent falls. In addition, beds that are easy to get in and out of are a good choice.

- *Child Safety Covers:* You should have safety covers on any door leading to the outside. The best ones are the locks that you can only open by entering a numeric code, because a dementia patient is unlikely to remember this code.

- *Child Safety Locks:* Not everything needs to be locked but you should lock up anything that can be hazardous to the patient. Medicine should be kept in a locked box; cleaning supplies should be in a locked cupboard and so on.

- *GPS Tracking Devices:* This was mentioned in wandering but having a tracking bracelet on the patient is important. If the patient wanders away from the house, it is easier to locate her.

- *First Aid Kit:* In case an accident does happen, it is important to have a well-stocked first aid kit in the home.

2. Infections

Since you can't see the microorganisms that cause most infections, you would be well advised to clean your house from top to bottom before your patient moves in.

In addition, make sure that you keep the house clean and avoid any homes if you know there is an illness going around.

If your patient does become ill, make sure that you follow the following tips to prevent secondary infections:

- Wear gloves whenever you come into contact with waste from the patient. Things such as disposing of faecal matter or laundering urine soaked clothes.

- Wear gloves only after washing your hands, and dispose of dirty gloves when you are about to touch clean areas.

- If the patient has an infectious illness, wash all surfaces or areas that may have been contaminated with body fluids, and wear a clean gown when performing personal tasks on the patient.

- Exercise particular care in handling needles, sharp objects, or contaminated material by wearing gloves and disposing of them in a special biohazard container. You can purchase them for the home if the patient needs frequent injections.

- Wash your hands frequently, particularly when in contact with body fluids, when preparing food or feeding the patient, and when touching the patient during toileting.

3. Falls
As I have mentioned many times in this book, falls are very common in patients with dementia, especially when they have Lewy Bodies dementia.

Patients are more likely to fall the older they are and the further their dementia has progressed. Falls are a risk because:

- With possible disorientation and being less steady on their feet they fall more frequently.

- Their bones are more brittle than younger people and will break more readily.

- They can get a fracture, such as a fractured or broken hip, and that can develop into more problems and, frequently, death.

117

To prevent falls, you should remove all clutter from the house. Pick up throw rugs and store them away. In addition, rearrange electric and telephone wires so that they are not in the way.

If steps in the house are uneven or you have sloping floors, contact a contractor to help fix those areas so the patient has more stability in those areas. If they cannot be fixed, section off those areas with baby gates to keep the patient from them. For areas that can't be sectioned off, use red tape to mark a hazard. This does not always work but it can help reduce the chances of a fall occurring.

- Another way to prevent falls is to improve the lighting wherever the patient might venture, including nightlights in passageways.

- Avoid cleaning materials that create slippery floors and use non-skid mats in areas where water could be, such as near entrances and in the bathroom. In the bathroom itself, install grab bars in the shower and tub and near the toilet.

Another area that poses risks results from disorientation, memory loss, balance issues, and medications that may cause drowsiness. Thus you would be well advised to be pro-active as follows:

- Avoid having the patient wear clothing that is too long and can impede walking.

- Keep eyeglasses and other frequently used items close to her so that she won't have to walk around to get these.

- Avoid waxing floors and use non-skid flooring materials wherever possible.

- Non-skid socks and non-skid shoes are advisable for the patient as well.

- Mop up or clean a spill as soon as you see it.

- Encourage trips to the bathroom.

- Lock the wheelchair when assisting the patient in and out of one or when stationary.

- Get walkers, canes or other accessories to reduce the risk of a fall.

- Use hardware-mounted gates at the top of stairs and safety gates wherever the patient may want to go.

4. Burns or scalding

Another common safety hazard that can occur in the home are burns. Burns can be caused by dry heat, such as a hot iron, stove, or a hot appliance; wet heat can be caused by boiling water or other liquids, or chemicals, such as certain acids. You can take the following steps to prevent burns and scalds:

- Ensure that the patient is sitting down before serving hot drinks.

- Hot drinks should be poured in a direction away from the patient, and hot drinks should be kept with a lid on and away from the edges of tables.

- Tell the patient that you are about to pour a hot liquid.

- Have the hot water heater altered and set at lower temperatures so tap water is not as hot.

- Run the cold water first, followed by the warm water, when running a bath.

- Always check water temperature with a thermometer or your wrist.

- Check that all appliances and the stove are off when you're not using them and before leaving the home.

- Faulty appliances are dangerous; if they look like they need repairing, put them away until they are repaired; put all appliances away after usage.

5. Choking, cuts, and poisoning

Dementia patients are commonly at a greater risk of choking as they frequently have difficulty chewing and swallowing. For this reason, it is very important to be aware of the possible choking hazards that can be around the house. Patients with dementia can cause self-harm so it is important to keep hazardous and/or dangerous items out of reach and safely locked away.

Some tips to follow are:

- Keep small items out of reach of the patient.

- Cut food into small morsels or puree it.

- Sharp objects in the bathroom or kitchen should be kept out of reach. These would include nail clippers, razors, knives, peelers, scissors, food processor blades and glass with sharp edges.

- Cleaning products should be kept in a locked cupboard.

- Glues and paints should be kept out of reach.

- Medications should always be kept in a locked box.

- The poison control number should always be kept handy. Number that you should know are:
- In the U.S. (1-800-222-1222)
- In the UK (0845 4647)

6. Fire hazards and Prevention

Fires are a dangerous hazard in the home of someone with dementia, and the stove is the number one culprit. Fires, however, can be caused by any of these:

- Smoking and careless disposal of lit buttes. The patient's home should really be a smoke-free environment, and you can enforce that with anyone who visits.

- Kerosene, gasoline and paint thinners are particularly flammable, so is natural oxygen gas, and spark producing equipment such as heaters and appliances.

- Old electrical wires and electrical outlets that visibly need replacing should be replaced.

- Choking off grills from their venting grills or registers, particularly those in sleeping areas.

- Heaters, or anything that can produce a spark or flame, left next to draperies, clothing, or other bedding or clothing fabrics can lead to a fire.

- The stove in the home. It is not uncommon for a patient to use a stove without realizing it. When you are not able to watch the patient, the stove should be unplugged.

Here are some other precautions you should take against fire hazards:

- Have a fire extinguisher in the kitchen placed in a location that you can get to in case the stove is on fire. Check the date when the extinguishers were last maintained and make sure it is in good working order, and that you know how to use it. If it has not been maintained, have it serviced or purchase a new one.

- Be sure there are working smoke alarms in all the rooms (replace batteries when needed).

- Do not leave the dryer on, or any other appliance, when you leave house.

- Turn off space heaters at night or when everyone leaves the house.

7. Finding Time for Yourself

Now that you have your house proofed and ready for your patient, it is time to look at your own lifestyle changes. Remember that when you bring a loved one into your home to care for her, or you move to the patient's home, you are changing your lifestyle significantly.

You will be faced with 24 hour care and it can become very easy to forget about your own care. Before you take any steps to move the patient in, take the time to meet with everyone in the immediate family.

Find out how they are going to help you so that you can have some time for yourself. The best set up is to have someone come in to cover weekends. This will make care very similar to live in home care, which we will go over in later chapters.

If you do not have outside supports, it is important to hire a respite caregiver to come in and take care of your loved one, even if it is for only a few hours per week.

Taking time for yourself will help you to cope with the challenges of caring for a patient with dementia and will ensure that you do not burn out too quickly.

Chapter 15. Aids and Devises for Care

Earlier in this book, I went over the many aids and tools that you will need to help your patient with the day-to-day tasks they are faced with. Some of the aids that I will go over in this chapter will help you as a family to overcome some of the fears that having a loved one with dementia creates.

As you know, there are hundreds of items out there that are designed to make dealing with dementia easier. It can be a bit overwhelming when you are trying to figure out exactly what you need. Let's face it, if you bought every product that was pushed on you, you would have a house full of junk.

For that reason, I am not going to go over every single thing that you can purchase. It is important to assess your own needs and the needs of your patient.

Some of my recommended aids that will help you and your patient are:

1. GPS Trackers

One of the first things that I tell people to purchase is a GPS tracker for their patient as soon as possible. Since wandering is a very real danger that people with dementia face, having a GPS tracker of some kind or another is very important.
A GPS tracker is simply wonderful : the patient carries a device with her and you, the carer, can see on your computer or mobile phone where she is.

While most people hesitate about having a GPS tracker for their parent or loved one, they have actually come a long way. At one time, GPS trackers were rather clumsy and bulky. It was difficult to find a way for a patient to carry it without the risk of the patient dropping the item.

Today, GPS trackers have become much smaller and many times, a patient is unaware that the tracking devices are on them. In fact, you can purchase a number of different devices that have GPS trackers built in, including: Cellphones, Computers, Pagers, Bracelets, Shoes.

One of the most interesting developments in GPS trackers is the fact that you can now find them in items such as watches and necklaces. The patient does not even have to be aware that there is a tracker on her body.

However, watches and necklaces, as well as the larger items such as a cell phone are not ideal as patients may pull the watches off or drop the cell phone.

Because of this, I strongly recommend that you purchase a GPS tracking device that can either be placed in a shoe or purchase shoes that have tracking devices. These are very new to the market but they have had a lot of success. The bonus is that most dementia patients will not take their shoes off when they are wandering so you don't have to worry as much about the item being dropped or lost.

If you are interested in using a GPS tracking system, contact a GPS tracking service to find a manufacturer. Some manufacturers of GPS Trackers for dementia patients and services that monitor them are:

- Track Jack Europe: www.trackjackeurope.com
- Home Technology Systems, Inc.: www.hometechsystems.com
- EM Finders: www.emfinders.com
- ADT – Companion Service: www.adt.com
- Senior Technologies, Inc.: www.seniortechnologies.com
- Vision Localization Systems: www.keruve.com
- RF Technologies, Inc: www.rft.com
- Locator Systems Corp: www.locatorsystemscorp.com
- Secure Care Products: www.securecare.com

- Care Electronics, Inc.: www.careelectronics.com
- Wherify: www.wherifywireless.com
- Powderhorn Industries, Inc.: www.powind.com
- Project Lifesaver: www.projectlifesaver.org
- Care Trak International, Inc: www.caretrak.com

2. Memory Aids

Memory aids are another item that I really feel a caregiver should purchase. These are devices that are used to give a patient clues for memory. There are a number of different types of memory aids but the ones that I am talking about are computers where photos and other memories can be stored.

The patient is able to use the computer, or tablet, and focus on memories that are being displayed. While it may not seem like a must have, these computers are designed to monitor when a patient is lingering on a picture. When this happens, the computer gives clues to help the patient remember the memory.

Memory aids allow the patient to remain grounded in the here and now. While a photo is usually from a past experience, it triggers a recollection that allows the patient to remember the present. There are several devices on the market; however, one that I am excited about is the MemeXerciser, http://www.cmu.edu/qolt/Research/projects/current-projects/cognitive-coach.html.

3. Date Clocks and Calendars

Although almost every house has a clock and a calendar, you should think about purchasing date clocks that have the time of day as well as the month, day of the week and calendar date prominently displayed.

Clocks are very important for a patient with dementia because many patients need to reorient themselves several times during the day. This is usually done in the morning or in the evening but at any time of the day, a patient may need to become reoriented. A date clock will provide this so make sure that you have several in the home. You can purchase them at many stores both in your area and online.

- Search Amazon for "Day Clock" to find one.
- http://alzmall.com/alzheimers-products

4. Programmed Phones

Another item that is a good choice for patients with dementia is a programmed phone. This allows the patient to be able to phone people without having to remember a phone number or look for it in their phone book. There are many programmable phones on the market but I recommend that you avoid the traditional phones where you write the name beside an assigned number. Having to read a name or remember which name goes with which speed dial can make it difficult for a patient with dementia. Instead, choose a phone that can be programmable and one that you can place a person's photo on the phone. This enables the patient with dementia to have more freedom and they will be able to call people when they want to and if they need help.

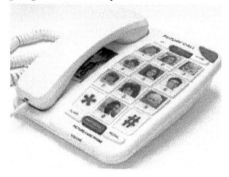

A good place to purchase photo phones is
http://alzmall.com/alzheimers-products/

5. Telecare Alarms

The final item that I feel is a must have for anyone who has dementia is telecare. These are devices that are set to sound an alarm if a particular event or emergency happens. The alarm lets the patient know when something is happening and it can also be tied into a caregiver's phone system or a monitoring system. What this means is that the device will call the caregiver immediately when something that has the potential to be hazardous occurs.

You can purchase telecare alarms for the following:

- *Flood Sensors:* These are sensors that are installed in the running boards and floors of a kitchen, bathroom or anywhere where there is a sink or running water. Many dementia patients will leave taps running and get distracted by other things. When there is a leak, an alarm will sound.

- *Gas:* While there are home alarms for various gases in the home, you can purchase a device to signal an alarm if the pilot light went out on a gas appliance or if the gas was left on. Another bonus is that you can also purchase a device that will shut off the gas as it gives the alarm.

- *Bed occupancy:* These are alarms that have a preset time limit on it. If a patient does not return to the bed after a set period of time through the night, an alarm will sound. In addition, the alarm will sound if the person does not get out of bed after an extended period.

- *Extreme Temperatures:* Many patients with dementia will have problems with temperatures in their home. They may turn up the heat during the summer or turn it off in the winter. You can purchase a device that will monitor the temperature in the home and will sound an alarm if there is an extreme shift in normal temperatures.

As you can see, many of the must have devices that I recommend revolve around safety. The reason for this is because it will not only keep your patient safe but will also give you peace of mind when you cannot be there for her.

http://alzmall.com/alzheimers-products/

Chapter 16. Caring for a Patient with Dementia

There is a lot to do to prepare yourself for when caring for your loved one with dementia. It is not a task that you should take lightly and it is something that will take up a large portion of your life. Caring for someone with dementia is more than simply creating the proper environment for her. It is all the little, day-to-day things that the person did on her own, which we will go over in this chapter.

1. Personal Care

The very first thing that you should consider with care is how you are going to assist your patient with their personal care. Personal care usually includes, but is not limited to, toileting, shaving, brushing hair and teeth and bathing. When the patient is in the early stages of dementia, there is not a lot that needs to be done, however, as the disease progresses; you will find that you need to take over most, if not all, of the personal care.

Administering Medication:

As a caregiver, it is your responsibility to properly dispense and administer the medication that has been prescribed.

You should never trust a patient to take her medication on her own, especially as her dementia progresses. Keep the medication in a locked cabinet. When you give the medication, make sure that you watch the patient to be sure that she takes it.

Shaving:

Shaving can be a difficult task for a caregiver as it can be a time when you need the patient to sit still. To shave a patient, explain to the patient what is going to be happening before you start. Continue explaining it as you shave the patient. For shaving, use safe tools to prevent injury. There are safety razors available or you can use an electric razor instead.

Daily Grooming:

If it is possible, it is important to encourage the patient to groom herself on a daily basis. This enables the patient to feel a sense of control over herself and her day and will give her feelings of accomplishment. You may need to help her with some tasks or with manipulating the tools but if she can do it on her own, allow her to. Remember, it doesn't have to be done perfectly when the patient does it herself.

Bathing:

Bathing is an intimate type of personal care that can be difficult for both the caregiver and the patient. A positive aspect of bathing is that the patient will feel better and refreshed when she's clean, which in turn is rewarding to you.

Before you bathe your patient, it is important to explain exactly what is going to happen. Go over the equipment that you are using as well before you use it. For example, I am going to scrub your skin with the washcloth. This will help reduce the stress that being bathed by someone else can cause.

Bathing is tricky and frequently results in accidents, particularly when the patient has dementia. People require bathing two or three times a week, sometimes even less; however, the patient will need genital areas washed on a daily basis.

Planning before bathing is of critical importance: plan the desired temperature when the patient is wet, plan the towels you are going to need and position them appropriately, plan every step you are about to embark on, and get your needs (shower stool, relaxing chair after the bath, clean clothes).

If you need to lift the patient, make sure you have the proper equipment in the bathroom to help you in that regard. When the patient is in the tub, never leave her alone, even for a few seconds, as an accident can happen very quickly.

Nail Care:

Nail care is important when it comes to dementia patients. Remember that there are some behaviours that can be self injurious and having long nails can lead to more injuries. Use child safe nail clippers to cut the nails and soak the nail before you fix cuticles. Never use a tool to push back a cuticle.

Dental Care:

Dental care, such as brushing the teeth and flossing, should be performed twice a day. The best time to do this is after breakfast and before bed, however, if the patient is prone to sundown dementia, it is better to do it after the last meal of the day. This will help cut down on the agitation.

Again, make sure that you clearly outline what is going to happen to the patient. This will make it much easier to do. If you can, have the patient brush her teeth on her own or assist her in manipulating the brush.

When you are brushing the teeth, check for ulcers or tiny, painful white sores. Also, make sure the patients tongue is not swollen or encrusted, and look out for possible infections or irritations. In addition, be alert to possible wobbly, fragmented or festered teeth, and chapped lips.

If she has dentures, handle them carefully and care for them by washing them in cold water daily and following the instructions that you were given by the denture specialist.

Toileting:

Like many of the personal care challenges, toileting may be something that the patient does on her own for much of the time you are caring for her. However, it is very common for incontinence to occur in the later stages of dementia and this should be taken into consideration.

At some stages of dementia, the patient may need to wear adult nappies as they are unable to make it to the bathroom. In other cases, the patient may be able to hold her bowel movements or bladder but may not have the mobility to use the bathroom without assistance.

From my own experience I can tell you that you need find a system to count the adult nappies. My grandmother used to tell me, when she was still reasonably well, that she had taken a new nappy every day. After a while I started to realise that the nappies didn't go down quick enough so I knew she was not using a fresh nappy daily, which was very important for her (and for anybody else as well) because she is prone to urine infections. That was an extra indication for my mum that grandmother could no longer live on her won to look after herself.

There are many ways to help a patient with toileting and these can be.

- *Using a bedpan:* This works better for men then it does for women but you can use a fracture pan for women. It should be slid under the patient so they can relieve themselves. Before you use it, warm the bedpan and add a small amount of baby powder to the edges to prevent it from sticking to the patient.

- *Portable Commode:* This is a toilet that can be used like a regular toilet. The only difference is that you will need to empty the commode when the patient is finished going to the bathroom. Be sure to help the patient on and off of the commode and don't leave them unsupervised.

- *Regular Bathroom:* Lastly, you can do toileting in the bathroom as you normally would. This only works if the patient is able to hold her bladder long enough to make it to the bathroom. You may need to help with lifting the patient on and off the toilet. Again, make sure you stay with the patient to avoid any accidents from happening.

When you are helping the patient with toileting, it is important to let them know what is happening. This can be a very difficult part of the day for a patient so it is important to really focus on making it as positive as possible.

2. Mobility Care

Another area of care that you will need to provide for your patient is mobility care. Again, the amount of mobility care that you need to provide will change depending on the stage of dementia that she is in. In the early stages, she may not need any help with mobility.

Transfers:

This refers to any type of movement for your patient when she needs to be lifted. This could be moving from the bed to the wheelchair or from the wheelchair to the toilet.

Safety is a major concern when you are doing transfers, as some patients may be heavy or tall. Many patients may have a "strong side" and may also be resistant to being transferred, so make sure that you move the patient from the strong side first. Also, make sure you lift with your legs to avoid injuring yourself during the transfer.

Before you move the patient, explain to her the procedures you are about to take, confirming, if possible, that she understands. Make sure the patient has non-skid slippers on. Be mindful of your own body alignment – if you can, have a physical therapist teach you how to execute the various types of transfers. Bend your knees, and lean forward against the patient. Ask her to lean against you. Circle her body firmly with your arms, bringing her as close to your body as possible, and then, on the count of three, stand her up.

This can be exhausting to both you and the patient so be sure to keep an eye on her stamina. Make sure you have a chair handy to provide her with a break whenever she needs a breather.

Positioning:

This is of particular importance for patients who are bed bound or spend a lot of time in bed. Being able to properly prop up the patient will help make the patient feel more comfortable and it can foster good health.

Use pillows to help position the patient and also make sure that you have bed cradles and hand rolls to help offer a range of positions.

With positioning, it is important that you change the position of the patient every two hours if they are unable to do it on their own. Every time that you change a position, rub the patient's back or limbs to help with circulation. In addition, take the time to check the patient's skin condition to make sure there are no bedsores.

Ambulating:

The word to ambulate means to walk, and although many patients with dementia can walk, they may be unsteady and in need of assistance. Make sure that you have the proper safety tools for your patient, such as gait belts, crutches, canes and walkers.

When you are walking with a patient with dementia, you should make sure that you walk half a step behind her on her left hand side, holding her left forehand and elbow firmly.

3. Nutritional Care

Another area of care that the caregiver will be in charge of is nutritional care. This is very important, because people with dementia are more likely to miss meals or forget to drink water during the day. A poor diet cannot only cause the dementia to progress faster but it can lead to other health problems.

It is important to speak to the patient's physician when you are planning a diet for her. There may be some health problems that can be affected negatively by the types of food that the patient eats. In addition, a plan with a trained dietician can make caring for your patient that much easier.

When you are planning meals for your patient, make sure you do the following:

- *Keep the meals small.* Remember that as we age, we tend to have a harder time with large meals. A patient with dementia is no different and she may lose focus on the meal if it is too large.

- *Plan for 6 meals instead of three.* Have 6 meals, and even up to 8, planned for a day. These meals will be smaller and will help keep her appetite up.

- *Have a set schedule for meals.* Always have a set schedule for the meals of the day. Do not expect her to eat whenever you get a chance.

- *Make the meals appealing.* This means that you should season it the way she likes and present it in an appealing way.

- *Offer ample water.* Water and other beverages are very important as dehydration can lead to outbursts and can also lead to health problems. 6 to 8 glasses of water should be given to the patient daily.

- *Remember her challenges.* Lastly, remember the challenges that eating may present. Does she have difficulty chewing? Do some foods disagree with her stomach? Make changes to the menu to help avoid these challenges.

If you think in these terms, meal planning does not have to be difficult, especially if you are under the guidance of a dietician. When your patient is eating, make sure that you are there to supervise it, in case of choking. In addition, make sure that you follow these tips:

- *Watch for discoloration.* Throughout the day, make sure that you watch for discoloration in the skin. This can tell you whether your patient is dehydrated or is not getting the proper nutrients.

- *Make sure she is sitting.* Always have your patient sitting for a meal. You may have to move her to a sturdy chair to accomplish this. If she is prone to wandering while eating, encourage her to stay sitting, as this will prevent her from losing interest in her meal. It will also prevent choking.

- *Mash the food.* If she is having a difficult time chewing or swallowing, make sure that you mash the food to ensure that she does not choke.

The key with meals is to keep it informal and enjoy the time with your patient. She will be more likely to eat if it is an enjoyable experience and it will give you some time to relax and bond with your loved one.

4. Daily Chores

When you take on the responsibility of a loved one with dementia, you often take over the responsibilities of the daily chores. It is important to remember that you will need to do all the cleaning in the home. This includes laundry and basic home maintenance.

You will also be in charge of the daily errands. Grocery shopping, filling prescriptions, scheduling medical appointments and banking are all errands that you will have to do on behalf of the patient.

Another role that you will have to fill is the role of communicator with the outside world. Make sure that you get out and communicate with family, friends and health professionals on how the patient is doing. Encourage your patient to come out when you are communicating with people, as it will help them be social, which is very important.

5. Companionship

The final type of care that you should provide your patient is companionship. As I have mentioned many times in managing behaviours and mood changes, dementia is an isolating disease. This means that they often feel disconnected from the outside world.

Providing companionship is a vital task that many patients yearn for. Make sure that you encourage conversation with your patient and be attentive to issues she may be facing like loneliness, isolation, withdrawal, and depression.

Don't pressure her into discussing her feelings if she does not want to. Remember that occasionally, she may not be able to communicate what is wrong and this can become worse as the dementia progresses.

While you will be the main source for her companionship, it is vital that you find other companionship for her. A pet in the home has been proven to be beneficial for dementia patients and will help prolong good health.

Other ways to provide companionship for the patient is to go out to social events and activities at senior centres. You can also attend shows and other events to keep her stimulated. Joining a walking club will provide her with exercise and is a social experience.

Make sure that whenever you take her out to these social events, you go with her to ensure that she stays safe the entire time.

Providing quality care can be challenging at times but by providing care, you will have ample opportunities to spend quality time with a person you love. So I strongly recommend that you look at the moments together as a blessing and that will make the journey through dementia much easier for both of you.

Chapter 17. Remedies for Dementia

Before we look at finding outside care for your loved one, I wanted to stop and look at the various different remedies that are out there for dementia. One thing that I want to stress is that dementia is not curable. It is a progressive disease and at this current time, they have not been able to find any cure for it.

There are many different medications that a doctor will prescribe to help reduce the effects of dementia. This will prolong the prognosis but not the gradual deterioration that is occurring.

When you are looking at remedies for your patient, it is very important to take those points into consideration. When I was looking to help my grandmother, I was surprised by the flood of natural remedies that are being marketed. While some look very promising, it is important to remember that all of these remedies are stop gaps. They will help reduce the effects and also the progression of the disease, but they are not an end all, be all cure.

Some of the remedies do not work at all so make sure you do your research on the remedy before you start using it. In this chapter, I will go over a few of the more popular remedies that people have been using with mixed results.

Please remember that none of these are proven methods and I suggested to do your own further investigation to see if any of these are suitable for your patient.

1. Coconut Oil

Over the last few years, there has been a major shift to more natural methods with dealing with dementia. One of these shifts have been towards looking at the benefits of coconut oil. Of all the remedies that are out there, I find that this one has the most benefit. It falls under a low risk but potentially high benefits category and I recommend that you try it to see if the symptoms of dementia do, in fact, lesson.

The main reason why I have said it like that is because dementia is not cured with coconut oil. In addition, it has surprising benefits for some patients with dementia but next to none for other patients.

Although studies are still being conducted on the effectiveness of coconut oil for a dementia patient, it is believed that the coconut oil affects the ketone levels in the body, which are used by the brain to function. When a patient eats coconut oil or has it added to her diet, her body begins producing higher levels of ketones and this leads to the brain being able to work properly.

In addition to reversing some of the symptoms of dementia, coconut oil is said to be an excellent preventative. Adding a few tablespoons to your daily diet will reduce the risks of developing dementia.

If you are planning on adding coconut oil to your patient's diet, make sure you check with her physician to ensure there will be no risks involved. You can also use coconut oil for cooking.

Next, give the patient 1 tablespoon of coconut oil directly, every day and then add a few extra teaspoons of coconut oil to her diet. Gradually increase the amount of coconut oil that she is eating until she is taking 2 tablespoons of coconut oil directly every day and she has a maximum of 3 tablespoons of coconut oil added to her diet.
http://coconutketones.blogspot.com.br
http://www.coconutketones.com/whatifcure.pdf
http://www.coconutketones.com/

2. Vitamin D and Vitamin D3

When we talk about diet, we often talk about the various vitamins and minerals that can be added to your diet as a supplement. Studies have shown us that vitamins and minerals play a very important role of staving off potential health problems and also for reducing the effects of some illnesses.

Vitamin D and vitamin D3 are two of those vitamins that have proven to have substantial benefits for anyone who takes supplements containing them. While studies are still being done on the long-term effects of vitamin D and vitamin D3 on dementia patients, there are studies that have shown it to be beneficial to reducing the effects and risks of cardiovascular diseases.

It is this correlation with cardiovascular remedies that has given doctors and many organizations that deal with dementia hope. While it may not affect all forms of dementia, it may have benefits in combating vascular dementia specifically.

There have been some studies that have shown that vitamin D and vitamin D3 reduce the symptoms of dementia. There have also been links that these vitamins slow the progression of the disease. However, more studies are being done to determine the exact benefits.

Regardless of whether the studies have been finished, one thing that is certain, is that vitamin D and vitamin D3 are important vitamins that boost our health and sense of well being.

It is very simple to give a patient a vitamin D supplement and you should try to give them 5000IU's per day.

3. Herbal Treatments

Another popular remedy for patients with dementia is herbs and various herbal remedies. When it comes to herbal remedies, there are some that really do work at prolonging periods of good health in dementia patients. However, it is very important to be realistic about the expectations that you have.

Most herbal treatments work well for one symptom but not for another. That is why a patient may need to use several different types of herbs to be sure that all the symptoms are treated.

While there is not always a problem, some herbs, when mixed together or mixed with medication, can have adverse effects on health. It is very important to speak with your patient's physician before you use any herbal remedies.

That being said, in the world of dementia care, there are two different herbs that are often viewed as an exception because there have been known benefits. These are Gingko and St. Johnswort.

Gingko is a plant that has been cultivated for thousands of years in China and is seen as a miracle plant. The main reason for this is because it is an antioxidant that aids in removing free radicals from the body.

Gingko has long been tied to benefiting dementia patients, as it has successfully delayed the progression of dementia. While it does not cure later stages of dementia, if it is administered in the early stages, it will prolong the quality of life that your loved one has.

St. Johnswort is another popular herb and it is believed to be effective for dementia patients as well. However, it is not because it delays dementia but because it often helps ease the symptoms of depression, which is very common in dementia patients.

Being able to have a brighter and happier mood helps promote health and enables the patient's own body to work against the progressive disease.

When St. Johnswort is combined with Gingko, the benefits are significant and the outlook is very good.

4. Magnetic Fields

The final treatment that I am going to mention is treating dementia through the use of magnetic fields. This is a treatment where the patient is exposed to low-level magnetic fields in an effort to repair the damage done to the brain.

While many feel that there is a benefit, extensive studies on magnetic fields have actually linked low exposure to a greater risk of dementia. With that in mind, it is hard to believe that something that may cause dementia is the best way to treat the symptoms.

The final thing that I want to leave you with in this chapter is the reminder that there are always the latest and greatest when it comes to remedies. Everyone says that they have found the next miracle cure and while it may work for some, the majority of cures are scams.

Make sure that with whatever remedy you begin looking at that you research it thoroughly. In addition, discuss it with the patient's doctor before you administer any type of alternate remedy. Some herbs react badly with some medications and it could lead to serious side effects including death.

Always follow the rule of thumb with remedies – if it is low risk but the potential benefits are high, then it is worth trying. If it doesn't work but there are no side effects, then you are no worse off than you were before you tried it. However, if it works, it will only improve the quality of life for your loved one.

5. A word about medication

I am not a doctor therefore I am not going to write a lot about medication. I can however tell you from experience and interviews that the following is very important.

- Whatever the doctor suggests, always investigate it further yourself. All medications have side effects. Make sure you are aware of all the side effects, before starting the medication.

- Don't ever stop medication without consulting your doctor.

- There are "white products" on the market. This means pills that are manufactured by another company, not the chemical company that launched the medication. My advice is not ever to buy those products, even if they are cheaper. There are mean people out there who pretend the medication is the same, just so they can profit. In reality, they often do not contain exactly the same ingredients as the original medication.

- Doctors these days often prescribe medication to try and stop the progress of dementia. According to studies, these do work but it is VERY important NEVER to stop these tablets all of a sudden as that might result in the patient going down VERY rapidly.
I have a friend who's mother was admitted to a care home. The care home stopped the medication from one day to the other, without consulting the family members. The decision was made simply for cost reasons. One month after my friend's mum went into the home, she didn't recognise any of her children, which she could do perfectly before she went into the home.

- ALWAYS, ALWAYS check that the medication is given correctly.

Chapter 18. Finding outside Care

Throughout this book, I have looked at providing care for your loved one on your own. In fact, many of the tips on how to manage aspects of dementia are to help you, the family member, manage.

It is important to take a step back from how you are going to help your parent, sibling, spouse or grandparent and look at what is best for him or her. Many times, dementia gets to the point where it becomes apparent that outside care or outside help is needed.

It is a decision that can leave many families feeling guilty and remorse but for those families and their loved one, it is the right choice. There is no right or wrong when it comes to this choice and it is important to do what is right for both you and your family.

In this chapter, I will go over seeking outside care and touch on both the different types of outside care and the costs that can be incurred.

The costs that I outline in this chapter reflect the costs that are found in the United States. For costs in the UK, read the chapter at the end of this book and for costs in other parts of the world, contact your local public health board.

I believe, from talking to people, that there is a shortage of care for dementia patients, almost everywhere.

Types of Outside Care

As you know, there are many different types of outside care that you can choose from for your patient. You can bring the care into your home or into the home of the patient. You can also place your patient into a home or institution. In this section, I will discuss many different areas on finding outside care including the type of care, the cost and tips on how to make this type of care work for you and your family.

1. Option One: In-Home Care

One of the most common forms of outside care for patients with dementia is in home care. This is where a caregiver will come into the home and will do a number of things with the patient. Care can include administering medication, bathing the patient, cooking meals and even taking the patient out to various appointments.

There are actually two different types of in-home caregivers you can hire – private caregivers, which are screened by you or agency caregivers, which are screened by an agency. There are pros and cons to both.

Private caregivers tend to be slightly less expensive; however, they do not always have the experience or knowledge needed. Agency caregivers usually hire trained and experienced caregivers; however, their costs are usually higher.

While the tips later on in this section will help you hire a private caregiver or one from an agency, I am going to focus primarily on agency caregivers since statistics and data is more current and available.

When you hire an agency caregiver for a patient, there is a very good chance that the caregiver will be certified in some way or another. Some certifications that you should look for are:

- CNA: Certified Nursing Assistant
- PCA: Personal Care Assistant
- HHA: Home Health Aide
- RN: Registered Nurse

While the last one is not always seen, many retired nurses looking for part time work when they retire will hire on with a care agency. The majority of agencies use CNA's, as they provide a wide range of services and have the knowledge needed to care for patients with dementia.

Regardless of the background that the caregiver has, they should have the following skills and criteria:
- Tested for tuberculosis
- Trained in CPR and Standard First Aid
- Certified in some form of home care
- Experienced with at least 120 hours in their field

Choosing an In-Home Care Agency

When you are looking for a caregiver, it is important to approach several different agencies. Do not choose the first one you pull from the phone book but take your time. Ask for advice from other people who use in home care or ask your physician for referrals.

After you have narrowed it down to a few agencies, contact them and let them know that you are looking for in-home care. Make sure that you give them full disclosure on the following:

- The diagnosis of the patient

- The days and times that you need care

- Symptoms of the patient

- The amount of supervision needed

- The extra work that will be involved in the care

It is very important to be completely honest for several reasons. One, you want your loved one to be cared for properly. Two, you do not want to lose a caregiver because you were not candid. Three, you do not want a new charge to be added to an already expensive care.

When you are choosing your agency, it is important to look at a few points. These are:

One: Is the agency busy?

Take the time to go into the agency that you are considering. When you get there, check to see how busy they are. Is the phone ringing? Do they have a full staff? If the answer is yes, then that should be a good indicator that they are sought after. In addition, you need to make sure that they are not too busy. You want to find one that is busy but not overwhelmed. If they are too busy, they may not have enough caregivers to provide quality care.

Two: How many caregivers do they have?

The best combination is a moderately busy agency with a wealth of caregivers for you to choose from. If they only have a few caregivers, then those caregivers may be stretched a little too thin. This can lead to a high turnover rate and may lead to improper care of your loved one.

Three: Do they show self-pride?

Another area to watch for is self-pride. Are they promoting their highlights when you go in or do they only talk about what they are going to offer? While you are in the office, listen to the incoming calls. Most calls are from caregivers –some on assignment checking in, others waiting for assignments- I would listen carefully to the receptionist's tone in dealing with those who at times sound desperate for lack of work. How the caregivers are handled by the receptionist is a reflection on the agency's culture. Are all the calls handled deferentially and with friendliness, or does the receptionist slip at times into impatience and condescension? For my loved one, I would want an agency that promotes self-esteem and respect, particularly with the down-trodden.

Four: How high is the turnover rate for caregivers?

One thing that you may notice when you are searching the agencies is that there is the same caregiver listed with more than one agency. This is completely normal since agencies often draw from the same pool of caregivers.

Caregivers, for the most part CNAs, or Certified Nursing Assistants, usually strive for three factors: first they want the patient to be close to where they live; then they want the assignment to have a schedule that matches their own; and finally they want a nice patient, someone appreciative.

I recommend that anyone looking for a caregiver meets the first two requirements. Find one that lives within 10 to 15 miles and one whose schedule meets your own. While your loved one may not be patient or appreciative, you can fill that requirement yourself to ensure that your caregiver does not go to a different job or agency.

Five: Does the agency provide proper screening?

Every state has different regulations regarding the screening of caregivers, so it is important to know the state regulations in your area. Generally, caregivers need to have criminal background checks, certifications verified, and references obtained. It is this latter requirement that has a lot of flexibility in it.

At some agencies, the Admin Assistant makes the calls to obtain the references, at others the Care Manager or Coordinator. If you are selecting a caregiver from an agency, ask to see the notes made by the administrator. In addition, ask if you can make a follow up call to the reference. This isn't always necessary but it can help fill in gaps in the report if you find it lacking in any way.

If the references are poor, even if the caregiver seems amazing, you should find a different caregiver. It is okay to ask for a different caregiver at an agency. If they say no, find a different agency.

Six: How does the agency react to emergencies?

Finally, check to see how the agency reacts to an emergency. Find out what precautions the agency has in place and how they deal with any problems.

For instance, if a patient has sundowner's syndrome and cannot be left unattended. She has continuous shift CNAs, 24 hours a day. It is the agency's responsibility to have the patient covered at all times. When someone doesn't show up, well, that's an emergency. A good agency will have resource to find other staff to fill in for the missing caregiver. This could either be other caregivers who have worked with the patient in the past or a number of caregivers who can easily fill in.

There are times when all that breaks down, and that's when the agency should be able to clearly identify what they would do next. What you want to know is that they always have responsible staff people on call that can be dispatched if an emergency does happen.

What does an Agency Offer

Although it may seem like a better option to go with a private caregiver since they are less expensive there are many things that an agency can do for you. Before we get into cost, I want to go over how agencies play a number of critical key roles.

- The agency takes care of the recruiting effort of caregivers on a daily basis, thus being able to maintain a large roster of caregivers, both live-out and live-in. These rosters allow for a wide range of caregivers with different levels of competence to suit every patient. This way, when you need a caregiver for your patient, and you tell them where she lives, they would have several caregivers to choose from who could go to that location. In addition, they will be able to choose within the guidelines you have given to match the caregiver's temperament that will mesh well with the patient.

- The agency selects the most suitable caregiver for the patient, based on your briefing.

- The agency is there to fill in when a caregiver is sick, or for weekends; when you hire an agency for 7-day live-in coverage, they undertake to have the patient covered all the time, without gaps. They understand that she cannot be left unattended – not even for a few minutes.

- The agency supervises their caregivers regularly by way of both their Care Coordinators who do the scheduling, as well as an RN who provides oversight on all assignments. The agency's task is to coach and mentor their caregivers constantly and make sure they abide by the governing policies and procedures at all times.

- The agency makes all payments to the caregivers, their daily commuting and other expenses, and their taxes when applicable, and the agency then bills you. In a sense, you would have outsourced all those money issues to the agency, thus avoiding having to make out-of-pocket payments on a frequent basis.

- The agency meets with other members of the "Care Team" that may be helping the patient. This includes other RN's, other medical staff, medical supply companies, and hospices. The caregivers are trained to be courteous and helpful when professional healthcare people from other organizations visit.

151

Cost of Hiring From an Agency

After you have found the agency and caregivers that you want caring for your loved one, it is time to start looking at the actual costs of this care.

When it comes to their rates, agencies usually retain a third or so of what you pay. The trend these days is for their caregivers to be hired as "1099" independent contractors, as against "W-2" employees, but you shouldn't have to be concerned with that.

For their share of the take, agencies perform vital tasks on your behalf: an RN provides insight over the patients wellbeing; a Care Manager staffs the patient's needs and supervises the caregiver on a day-to-day basis, changing her should a problem come up; they fill in on weekends or when the caregiver is sick; and they handle all payments to the caregiver.

When dealing with an agency, you should receive an invoice. You don't have to worry about work eligibility or taxes - you outsource all that to the agency.

The actual cost of the care differs depending on where you live and the type of care that is being given. If the care is only a few hours per week, the agency will usually set up a weekly fee or hourly fee for you. If it is all day, several days a week, the agency will usually have a daily fee, which is actually much cheaper than an hourly rate.

The costs that you can expect are:

- *2 to 6 hours of care per day:* Usually, the rate is set on an hourly rate for small periods of care. The average cost in 2012 is $16/hour; however, it can range from $14 to $20/hour.

- *6 to 8 hours of care per day:* This is an average work day and the caregiver will come during the day. Agencies usually charge a daily rate for the full day, even if you only need one or two days covered. The average rate for 2012 is $96/day (roughly $2900/month).

- 24 hours of care per day: If full care is needed, 24 hours per day, the cost goes up significantly to an average of $160/day ($4,800/month, or roughly $57,000/year).

Cost of Hiring a Private Caregiver

One thing that every family should know, is that there is a slight difference in cost between hiring an agency and hiring a private caregiver. Generally, the cost is less than if you were to hire an agency. It is important to note that when you do hire a private caregiver that there may not be any backups for emergencies, such as the caregiver is not able to go due to an illness.

In addition, you will need to pay the caregiver weekly and will need to find suitable arrangements for holidays and vacation days that the caregiver is entitled to.

Like agencies, you can hire a private caregiver for several hours or for entire days, up to 24 hour care. The average costs are as follows:

- 2 to 6 hours of care per day: Usually the rate is set on an hourly rate for small periods of care. The average cost in 2012 is $9/hour; however, it can range from $7 to $16/hour.

- 24 hours of care per day: If full care is needed 24 hours per day, the cost goes up significantly to an average of $90/day ($2,700/month, or roughly $32,000/year).

2. Option Two: Live-In Care

The second option that is available to families is a live-in caregiver. This is a person who moves into the home of the patient and provides 24 hour care. Like regular home care, a caregiver can be hired both privately and through an agency. The process of hiring, as well, is the same as for hiring an in-home caregiver.

As we look at the different options, live-in care that is offered 7 days a week, 24 hours a day is one of the more popular options for families. It gives them the security they need in knowing that their loved one is being taken care of properly. It also gives them a sense of peace because their loved one is in their own home.

While private caregivers can be hired, this is a bit of a struggle. For one, you have to go through the screening process yourself. For two, you have to be the one to fill in if the caregiver needs a day off or you will have to hire two caregivers. Finally, there is often a high turnover rate for live-in caregivers so you will often find yourself scrambling to replace the care. The problem with this is that, when your carer decides to leave, you could find yourself in a difficult situation as you will have to turn your life upside down again to look after the patient, whilst you are finding a replacement. If you work with an agency, should the carer leave unexpectedly, the agency will replace the carer immediately.

Agencies, on the other hand, take a great deal of pride in having good resources in place for live-in care, which includes a vast roster of live-in caregivers.

If you are not familiar with how a live-in caregiver works, the first step is to introduce the patient to the "primary" caregiver. This is the person who will live with the client from Sunday afternoon until Friday evening. The days may vary but this is usually the standard arrangement.

The main thing that they are looking for is for the patient to have a rapport with the caregiver. This will help minimize the stress the patient has when they see someone new in their home. When they have introduced everyone and you feel comfortable with the choice, the live-in caregiver will move into the home.

Although the focus is primarily on the main caregiver, the agency will also arrange introductions to any staff that will cover the "primary" caregiver. This will be whenever there is an emergency or during the weekends when the caregiver has her days off.

Generally, the secondary caregiver will arrive on Friday afternoon and stay with the patient until Sunday afternoon when the primary caregiver returns.

While the "primary" caregiver is usually consistent without many changes, it is typical that the agency will hire more than one secondary caregiver to cover a particular patient who will be able to fill in for the primary caregiver when necessary.

When it comes to live in care, there are three important benefits that families can experience.

- It is the least expensive way of providing around-the-clock coverage; it costs less than half of the cost of providing 24 hour services by way of two 12 hour shift personnel.

- It avoids the commotion of shift personnel coming and going every 12 hours; the tranquil atmosphere that it creates in the house is ideal for sundowning patients.

- The program is perfect for bonding between the caregiver and the care recipient; the two of them being together, conducting activities of daily living day and night.

Choosing a Live-In Caregiver

As I have already mentioned, choosing a live-in caregiver is exactly the same as choosing an in-home caregiver. Please read the section on finding out how to properly select an agency and what to look for.

In addition to those tips, it is important to ask the following questions before you move a caregiver into your loved one's home.

Q. What type of background should a caregiver have?

A. Caregivers can have a wide range of backgrounds and for many patients; their background can be anything from a nurse to a homemaker. However, when you have a patient with dementia, you want to have a caregiver that has significant experience with dementia.

In addition, you should hire a caregiver that has her HHA – Home Health Aide certificate. This will mean that the caregiver is trained in all the tasks needed for excellent medical and emotional care while still being able to provide a warm and loving service.

Q. What type of background check should I ask for?

A. Background checks are very important, especially when the caregiver will be living in the home with the patient. Make sure that they have criminal background checks and that they are bondable. In addition, always check the references. If there is an agency, the agency will do due diligence in this matter but do not hesitate to ask for copies of your own.

Other things that you want to check are verifications of certification and education. Past employers references, and if it is possible a skills test, to ensure that she can administer medication and do any other task the patient needs should be looked at.

Q. What other criteria should the caregiver have?

A. In addition to having her HHA certificate, you also want to make sure that she has an updated and current CPR and First Aid certificate. Vaccinations are also important and you want to confirm that she has had her TB vaccinations. If anything is not done, avoid hiring the caregiver until it is or look for another caregiver. Again, if you are going through an agency, they will make sure all of these things are done prior to the first meeting.

Regardless of whether you are hiring the caregiver yourself or working with an agency, it is important that you mesh with your caregiver. If you don't, ask for a different caregiver or look for a different one. Remember, you want to feel secure knowing that your loved one is being taken care of and if you don't like the caregiver or feel her skills are lacking, you will never have that piece of mind.

Cost of Hiring a Live-In Caregiver

The cost of hiring a live-in caregiver is not that much different than the cost of hiring 24 hour care. There is a flat rate for each day of care and if you have 7 days of care, it can become a bit expensive.

One thing that should be mentioned with live-in care is that the cost of food needs to be negotiated. Since many live in caregivers only keep a residence at the patient's home, they have lower overheads to maintain their residence. For that reason, it is important to work out the rate according to whether they will be eating with the patient or making their own meals and also if they will be returning to the house on their days off because they live there.

Room and board should be factored in and this can help reduce the price that is charged for daily care.

Another fact that needs to be factored in is the level of care that needs to be given. If you are asking for live-in care for a patient in early stages of dementia, then the care is usually minimum and is more of a companion role. However, if it is in the later stages of dementia, it can involve heavy lifting, managing medications and dealing with aggression and other behavioural, mood and medical problems. The more care that is required, the higher the cost will be for the live-in care.

Despite these different variables, the average cost of live in care is usually between $155 to $175/day or $57,000 to $64,000/year. Again, this can differ on different sides of the scale and it is not unheard of to spend upwards of $200 to $250/day for care. Private live-in care may be slightly lower but usually, the difference between private live-in care and agency provided live-in care is minor.

3. Option Three: Nursing Home Care

Nursing home care can be a range of different care options, from long-term care facilities, group homes, retirement homes or even assisted living. There is no right or wrong facility for you to choose from and it is important to assess the needs of the patient over the desires of the family. The reason why I stress this is because many families feel an obligation to keep the patient at home, even when it is clear that it cannot be done. It is important for the patient to get the best care possible and many times, that care is in an institution.

Many times, when families are faced with the choice of placing a family member into a home, it is due to a catastrophic event. The patient may have been hurt, become lost or may have had a frightening episode in the home. This has prompted a need to place the patient into a home and usually it is done very quickly, leaving families feeling completely overwhelmed.

It is important, however, that you try to take your time with finding a suitable care facility for your loved one. You may need to take a few days off or hire some respite care but the more time you spend looking, the better you will feel about your choice.

Choosing an Nursing Home

When the time comes to choose a nursing home, it is important that you involve everyone in the immediate family. If you are the person who will make the final decision, it is still important for everyone to share their feelings of a facility.

In the end, however, you will need to make the decision so your loved one can have the proper care and support that she needs. To choose a nursing home, it is important to follow these steps.

Step One: Decide on the Budget

Before you move forward and choose a nursing home, go over the budget to determine what you can afford. This is very important because many times, the nursing home is chosen with emotion. This leads to families getting in over their heads on a home that is much too expensive over the long-term.
If there are several family members who are going to share the cost of the nursing home, make sure you have several meetings on the actual cost. If the loved one will be funding her own care, be honest about her finances. This will prevent a lot of heartache down the road.
Later on in this chapter, I will touch on the costs of different forms of care.

Step Two: Determine the Needs of the Patient

Once you have the budget figured out, it is time to sit down and be honest about the needs of your loved one. Depending on the stage of dementia that your loved one is experiencing, you may have to have complete care or just assisted care.

It is important to really look at the care honestly and to plan for the future. There are many homes that offer a variety of assisted living and full care. The reason for this is that the transition to the full care facility is much easier when it is in the same home.

Step Three: Visit the Facilities

Before you decide on a nursing home, go to several different facilities to see what they have to offer. You want to make sure that the facilities are clean and cheerful. Also, make sure that there are enough staff to meet the needs of all the residents. Ask about hiring practices, if the staff have had criminal background checks and also what education backgrounds they have. The more information that you get, the better you will feel about your final choice.

When you are visiting, be sure to tell the facility the type of care your loved one needs. Don't lie or avoid the hard facts. Some facilities are not prepared to care for patients with dementia and it could lead to the services being revoked, which is something you do not want to happen.

Ask lots of questions and try to think ahead. Remember that dementia is a progressive disease so you want to make sure that you have the right information to plan for future care.

Step Four: Discuss the Options

After you have visited, take the time with the immediate family to discuss the options that you have. Take into account the cost, the services that are offered and the quality of the nursing home. When you feel comfortable with your choice, fill out the paperwork as a family.

Step Five: Follow Up

The last step is to follow up with the nursing home on a regular basis. Drop in when you can and ask to stay during the meal times. You want to go and see how your loved one is doing in the home. You also need to see if the care is as good as you believed it was.

If you have doubt about the care or treatment of your loved one at any time, make sure that you discuss those worries with the facility director, the patient's physician and other members of the care team. If things are not resolved, find a different home for your loved one.

Cost of a Nursing Home

The cost of a nursing home can differ depending on the amount of care that is needed and also the type of living arrangement. In addition, whether you have a private room or a shared room will change the cost.

Generally, you are looking at the following costs for a nursing home:

- *Assisted Living Facility:* The cost is at the minimum of $4,500 a month ($54,000/year), inclusive with heat and hydro paid for, as well as the assistance that is needed. Assistance does not include full time care and there may be hidden charges.

- *Nursing Home with Private Room:* Again, the cost can go up or down depending on the amount of assistance and the quality of the nursing home. The national average daily rate for a private room in a nursing home is $250, or $90,000+ a year.

- *Medicaid Nursing Home:* Medicaid is the state funded nursing homes that are reserved for patients that have a net worth of $4,000 or less. The facilities are usually lower quality and the care is not as good as other nursing homes. The cost is free, as long as the net worth is below $4,000 but it can cost several thousand a month if the net worth is too high.

In the end, it is important to decide on the type of care that works for your family and your loved one. While cost does play an important role in the decision, the actual care your loved one needs should play a greater role, since some forms of care, such as assisted living, may be out of the picture due to her health and the stage of dementia she is in.

Chapter 19. What you can do to help

Whatever decision you have taken to care for the patient, here are a few things that you can do to help her, whether she lives at her home, in your home or in a residential home.

- Pretend all is fine. When speaking to a dementia patient, I think it is best to always pretend all is fine, nothing has changed compared to before the time she was a dementia patient. To explain further what I mean,
I have seen many family members shouting at the patient saying :
"You've asked me that 10 times already! " or
" Do you not remember anything?" or
" I've just told you that!" or
" Don't you even remember your own daughter's name!"

 This will make the patient agitated and angry and soon she will not be prepared to say anything out of fear of being shouted at. The best thing to do is just answer her questions again, as if it is the first time she asked it, even if she asked it 7 times before. That way, you can keep conversation and the patient will feel better as you appear to just answer her questions.

- Mental stimulation. It has been proven that mental stimulation can slow down the progress of dementia.
Try and encourage your patient (if this is still possible) to do crosswords, a puzzle, knitting, a simple quiz, reading a newspaper, listen to the radio, play a board game, gardening, word games, pay an instrument, etc...

- Make her surroundings safe. Implement some of the safety advice from this book to make sure her surroundings are safe therefore reducing accidents.

- Look at old photographs together. This will bring back memories and is usually very enjoyable for all parties involved.

- Check on a regular basis that the medicine is given correctly, even if it is given by professional people. Everybody makes mistakes! It is crucially important to double check.

- Make sure you check on a regular basis that the patient is eating enough and drinking enough fluids.
- Make time to listen and chat on a regular basis
- Show affection
- Make sure her privacy is respected. If at all possible, give her some hours of privacy.
- Make them feel good about themselves. Don't always moan and groan about silly not important issues.
- Try to understand how she feels.
- If possible, involve them with choices.
- Make sure they know they still have an important role to play in your life and other people's lives.
- Treat the patient with respect and dignity.

Remember: each dementia patient is a unique individual with their own background and experience of life. They all have different feelings, likes and dislikes. Dementia affects each person in totally different ways.

Chapter 20. UK Options and Costs for Dementia Care

As I mentioned at the beginning of this book, much of the care and costs of care look at North American costs or specifically at US costs. In addition, many of the statistics are also geared toward the US but dementia is a worldwide disease that affects millions of families every year.

For that reason, I want to finish this book by providing you with statistics on dementia as it affects the UK and the costs that family members and caregivers will experience.

1. Demographics in the UK

When it comes to the aging population, there are many common traits between U.S. and UK. In fact, the boomer generation is, in essence, exactly the same between both nations. There is a rapidly aging population and this population will revolutionize what it means to be a senior citizen because their attitudes are so different to those of their parents.

Market research contends that they are likely to be demanding and imaginative consumers of both products and services, seeking out information for themselves and refusing to be defined by their age group.

But even before the bulk of the boomers retire, lingering stereotypes of the average senior citizen as a frail and passive creature are already out of date.

Much like in the U.S., the senior sector of the community in the UK is in the midst of a dramatic and unprecedented demographic shift, with the number of young people dwindling.

People are living longer, having fewer children and are leading more active lifestyles, which ensure a longer period in the workforce. In addition, the baby boomer generation is a large chunk of the world's demographic and while many boomers are just entering retirement, this population base is aging rapidly. With age comes many health problems such as dementia.

Statistically, there are over 850,000 people living with some form of dementia in the UK. While the number of cases seems fairly small, when you look at the population base of the UK, the number is high. In fact, it is comparable to the 5.8 million people in the US who are living with dementia.

In addition, the majority of those 850,000 people diagnosed with dementia, only 15,000 patients are under the age of 65. What this means is that dementia is a disease that affects people during their golden years and it can be a long-term illness that taxes both the family and the patient.

There is also evidence to suggest that not only are people living longer in the UK, they are also staying healthier until an older age. This is referred to by health experts as "compression of morbidity," which means that a vast majority of UK citizens will experience a serious age related illness over their lifetime. Illnesses, such as dementia, that will need extended care by either families or medical staff.

While the problem may not seem large, the disparity between the young working population and its ever expanding population of senior citizens on entitlement benefits is causing concern on both sides of the Atlantic. Fewer working young are subsidizing a greater number of retired people leading to increased pressures on the governments in first world countries to increase the age of retirement.

With the chance of dementia increasing in our aging population, many families are thrown into complete turmoil as they try to deal with both the emotional turmoil the disease brings to a family and the financial burden.

2. Cost of Care in the UK

When a family is faced with a loved one suffering from dementia, they are faced with several different terms, including the term "Means testing." This is a term that is used to describe the patient's worth to determine how much aid can be offered from the government. The lower the patient's net worth is, the more services are offered by the UK government.

While this may not seem like the big problem when faced with dementia, it is actually one of the biggest a family will face outside of the medical problems. Finding the proper supports is a costly endeavour and finding out what services are covered by government funding can be a harrowing journey.

One obstacle that families face is that as our population ages, the number of seniors who own their own homes increases. This leads to more seniors failing the means test and subsidized care is denied. Families are left struggling to pay for the care themselves and it can lead to many different problems for the family.

Due to this, a staggering number of homes are sold each year to cover the cost of providing care for patients with dementia. In fact, an estimated 70,000 homes are sold each year in the UK alone and families are left facing one of the largest financial commitments of their life – paying care fees – without any advice.

In fact the most recent research has shown that whether you are being funded by the State or paying privately for your care, it is important to have professional guidance on the programs out there. By having a knowledgeable support, you will be able to find the programs that you are rightfully entitled to. These programs are set up through a number of local authority or NHS or welfare benefits.

There are also specially designed financial products that can help meet the shortfall in income to cover the cost of care at the outset, often requiring just a part of your capital to be utilized to meet care costs, releasing the remainder for the eventual inheritance that so many older people wish to leave.

Contact Saga for further advice specific to your needs, call 0800 056 7996 or visit www.carehome.co.uk/fees/fees_advice.cfm for more information on the services that will help find the services and programs designed to make the cost of caring for a loved one with dementia easier.

The basic principle for the provision of community care is set out in the Government's "White Paper" called *Caring for People*. It states that "anyone who needs health or social care because of problems associated with old age; mental illness or learning, physical or sensory disabilities should be able to obtain care services and support, tailored to their individual needs whether at home or in residential accommodation."

One thing that is certain is that when a family is dealing with dementia, their focus should be on their loved ones. People should not have to seek out services and try to find the service that fits for them. Instead, there should be a service that enables families to be informed quickly and signed up to the programs even faster. Again, *SAGA* is a good place to start, as they will have access to many of the services you will need.

It is important to note; however, that you are entitled to an assessment regardless of whether your care is going to be State funded or paid for privately. As a private funder, it is particularly useful to have an assessment of your needs if there is a chance that your financial resources might reduce to the level where you would be seeking funding from the council in the future.

Again, the services and programs being offered are different from family to family and it is something that should be discussed privately with the members of your support team.

3. Frequently Asked Questions (FAQs) Regarding Costs

The values quoted hereunder apply mostly to England only. Wales, Northern Ireland and Scotland pay different amounts. It is important to note that these are estimates and the actual cost of care can differ depending on the severity of the dementia and the services required. Costs are estimates at the time of writing.

When helping a loved one move into a care home, it is important to understand what the State provides so you are certain about costs and affordability. Choosing care that will be unaffordable for you in the future can lead to more hardships for your family and your loved one.

To clarify some points on costs, below are a number of frequently asked questions and answers.

Q. Who qualifies for local authority financial assistance?

A. Qualifying can differ depending on the cost of living and the amount of income that you make. Generally, if you have a net worth that is below £23,250, you should be entitled to partial financial support from your local authority. If you have capital below £14,250 you will be entitled to maximum support, although you will still contribute to the payment, usually less than £22.30 per week, which will be retained for personal expenses.

If you have capital between £14,250 and £23,250 you will also pay a capital tariff of £1 per week for each £250 or part thereof between these two figures.

Q. If the state is paying; do I have a choice of care in a home?

A. Yes, even if the state is paying, you do have a choice of care at home, even if that care is in a different county. The home you choose must be suitable for your assessed needs, comply with any terms and conditions set by the authority and, not cost any more than they would usually pay for someone with your needs.

Q. What if the home costs are more than the local authority is prepared to pay for?

A. The local authority will allow the fees to be topped up by a third party who is able to do so over the long-term. You are not allowed to top up the fees yourself if you have an income of below £23,250.

Q. What if my partner needs care? Does that affect my own finances?

A. When you are looking at financial services regarding a partner, it is important to be aware that only the partner requiring care is subjected to the means test. Any property shared between the partners is disregarded if the partner is currently living in the properly. In addition, any savings or pensions that the partners share are only subjected to having 50% taken into account during a means test. What this means is that half of your shared net worth will be assessed and will affect the chance of financial support.

To help make the process easier, it is better to separate your finances into individual accounts before you go for the means test. This will not only ensure that your partner is assessed fairly but also that the process of assessment takes less time.

Q. What if I am funding my own care?

A. Although self funding is an option that many people diagnosed with dementia are faced with, it is important to understand your rights. Generally, self funded care is not eligible for any local authority funding. However, there are some financial services and assistance offered to those who self fund for their care. Make sure that you contact your local services to find out what programs can work for you.

Q. Will Social Services pay my fees while I am selling my former home?

A. If you have to sell your property to help pay for your care and you earn below £23,250, then the answer is yes, the local authority or social services will help pay your fees for up to 12 weeks of permanent care. After that point, if your home has not been sold, any fees paid by the local authority will be owing and will be recovered when your home does sell.

Q. Do I have to sell my property?

A. No, Social Services can lend you the money to pay for your care charged against your property value. However, they may limit how much they will pay and it could adversely affect your welfare benefit entitlements.

Q. Do I have to pay council tax on an empty property?

A. If you move into a care home and your property is left empty then you should receive full exemption from Council Tax until it's sold. Again, make sure you speak with a lawyer to make sure that your home is exempt.

Q. Is there any financial help that is not means tested?

A. If you are self-funding, Attendance Allowance is a non-means tested, non-taxable allowance paid at the lower rate of £47.80 per week for those needing care by day or night and, at a higher rate of £71.40 per week for those needing care by day and night.

In addition, whether your stay is temporary or permanent, if you receive nursing care in a care home you may be entitled to an NHS Registered Nursing Care Contribution (RNCC) toward the cost of your nursing care. When applicable, an amount of £108.70 per week is paid by the NHS directly to the nursing home as a contribution toward the weekly fees.

Another fund that you may be entitled to, if your needs are primarily health care needs, is full funding from your local Primary Care Trust (PCT). An assessment will need to be done according to their continuing care eligibility criteria before you can qualify for this funding.

Q. What happens if I move into a care home independently and run out of money?

A. This is a question that many families have since the reality of low funds is always present. Generally, when your capital is below, either initially or falling below, £23,250 you can seek local authority assistance. However, if the home costs more than the local authority usually pays and won't reduce its fees, you could be in the difficult situation of either finding a source to help pay for the difference in regards to care or finding a less expensive accommodation.

If there is a likelihood of running out of money, it is important for you to arrange an assessment of your care needs with the local social services department to ensure they will step in to help.

It is important that you contact Saga for any further advice that could pertain specifically to your case. They can be reached at 0800 056 7996.

4. Care at Home

When it comes to caring for a patient with dementia, regardless of the country you live in, there is an option to care for your loved one at home. In fact, many of the points through this book are designed to help you do this.

Before we close the book, it is important to understand that the cost of care, especially home care can be quite high. Although you may not require daily care for your patient, you will need some care on days when you cannot be with the patient.

The average cost for a private caregiver to come into your home is between £8 -£10/hour with some areas being more expensive. Remember that this rate is usually for a caregiver that does not have a significant amount of experience caring for patients with dementia.

If you are looking to hire a professional caregiver that has the credentials and experience needed to properly care for your loved one the rate you are looking at ranges between £12 - £16/hour. Again, this cost depends entirely on the caregiver's qualifications and other criteria, such as her experience with dementia.

The best approach in the UK in view of the high cost of hiring strangers is to try and find an accommodation with a neighbour or family member.

Chapter 21. Resources and References

In this section of the book, I wanted to leave you with a number of references and resources that will help you find enough information on both dementia and caring for a loved one with dementia.

It is important to find support in your own community. Your patient's physician is one of the best places to start, as they will have a list of services that are available close to you.

1. Family Support Resources

These resources are recommended for families that are caring for their loved ones themselves. It enables you to provide the care your loved one needs while maintaining their safety.

Safety Resources:
www.ext.colostate.edu
www.learnnottofall.com
www.safekids.org
www.webmd.com
www.startrightstarthere.com

Equipment Resources:
www.activeforever.com

www.seniorssuperstores.com

www.medicalguardian.com

2. U.S. Specific Care Resources

These services will help you locate the proper type of care for your loved one. It is an excellent place to get started and they can often direct you to services in your area.

Caregiver Resources:
www.completelongtermcare.com
www.assistedlivingamerica.org
www.housingcare.org
www.statistics.gov.uk

Funding Services:
www.medicaid.gov/

Referral Services:
www.carehomefinders.com
www.careproviderusa.com
www.visitingangels.com
www.elderlink.org

3. UK Specific Care Resources

As you know, there are a number of different services available to UK residents. It is important for families to look in their specific area. Below are a few organizations that will help get you started.

Saga:
www.carehome.co.uk

Referral Services:
www.independentreferralservice.co.uk
www.argyll-bute.gov.uk
www.bupa.co.uk
www.clinicom.cpft.nhs.uk

Support Services:
www.carersuk.org
www.counselling-directory.org.uk

Professional Supports:
www.crossroads.org.uk
www.scotland.gov.uk
www.dh.gov.uk
www.lifecoach-directory.org.uk

NHS and PCT services:
www.liverpoollifehouse.org
www.lcr.nhs.uk
www.nice.org.uk
www.nhs.uk
www.centrallancashire.nhs.uk

Respite Care and In-Home Care Services:
www.vitalise.org.uk/
www.agecare.org.uk
www.cedarscaregroup.co.uk/
www.korcare.co.uk
www.seniorcare24.be (for Belgium and Holland)

4. References

Below are a number of links that will provide more insight into caring for a patient with dementia.

www.caregiver.org
www.helpguide.org
www.dementiacentre.com
www.ageuk.org.uk
www.mayoclinic.com
www.emedicinehealth.com
www.ncbi.nlm.nih.gov
www.medicinenet.com
www.alz.org

www.emedicinehealth.com
www337.pair.com
www.lewybodydementia.org/
www.sciencedaily.com
www.alznyc.org
www.alzinfo.org
www.ncbi.nlm.nih.gov
www.indexmundi.com
www.prcdc.org
http://www.jfponline.com
http://www.alzheimers.org.uk
http://www.betterhealth.vic.gov.au
http://www.alzheimer-europe.org
http://www.helpguide.org
http://www.lewybodydementia.org
http://www.betterhealth.vic.gov.au
http://sundownerfacts.com
http://www.alznyc.org/caregivers
http://mom-and-dad-care.com
http://www.lewybodydementia.org

Lightning Source UK Ltd.
Milton Keynes UK
UKHW020630130121
376916UK00010B/2053